KU-299-526

Understanding Sexual Health

Editor: Tracy Biram

Volume 379

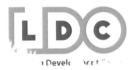 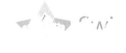

20 19003 725

NEW COLLEGE, SWINDON

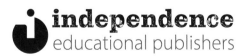
independence
educational publishers

First published by Independence Educational Publishers

The Studio, High Green

Great Shelford

Cambridge CB22 5EG

England

© Independence 2020

Copyright

This book is sold subject to the condition that it shall not,
by way of trade or otherwise, be lent, resold, hired out or otherwise
circulated in any form of binding or cover other than that in which it
is published without the publisher's prior consent.

Photocopy licence

The material in this book is protected by copyright. However, the
purchaser is free to make multiple copies of particular articles for instructional
purposes for immediate use within the purchasing institution.
Making copies of the entire book is not permitted.

ISBN-13: 978 1 86168 836 1

Printed in Great Britain

Zenith Print Group

Contents

Introduction

Understanding Sexual Health is Volume 379 in the **issues** series. The aim of the series is to offer current, diverse information about important issues in our world, from a UK perspective.

ABOUT Understanding Sexual Health

Sexual health is an issue that will always need open and honest discussion. This book explores the myths, facts and latest statistics on traditional topics such as contraception and STI prevention. It also looks at the importance of healthy, respectful relationships and examines the importance of more topical issues such as consent, sexting and safe online dating.

OUR SOURCES

Titles in the **issues** series are designed to function as educational resource books, providing a balanced overview of a specific subject.

The information in our books is comprised of facts, articles and opinions from many different sources, including:

♦ Newspaper reports and opinion pieces

♦ Website factsheets

♦ Magazine and journal articles

♦ Statistics and surveys

♦ Government reports

♦ Literature from special interest groups.

A NOTE ON CRITICAL EVALUATION

Because the information reprinted here is from a number of different sources, readers should bear in mind the origin of the text and whether the source is likely to have a particular bias when presenting information (or when conducting their research). It is hoped that, as you read about the many aspects of the issues explored in this book, you will critically evaluate the information presented.

It is important that you decide whether you are being presented with facts or opinions. Does the writer give a biased or unbiased report? If an opinion is being expressed, do you agree with the writer? Is there potential bias to the 'facts' or statistics behind an article?

ASSIGNMENTS

In the back of this book, you will find a selection of assignments designed to help you engage with the articles you have been reading and to explore your own opinions. Some tasks will take longer than others and there is a mixture of design, writing and research-based activities that you can complete alone or in a group.

FURTHER RESEARCH

At the end of each article we have listed its source and a website that you can visit if you would like to conduct your own research. Please remember to critically evaluate any sources that you consult and consider whether the information you are viewing is accurate and unbiased.

Useful Websites

www.ageuk.org.uk

www.better2know.co.uk

www.bishuk.com

www.brook.org.uk

www.disrespectnobody.co.uk

www.healthforteens.co.uk

www.healthyrespect.co.uk

www.independent.co.uk

www.news-decoder.com

www.nhs.uk

www.publichealthmatters.blog.gov.uk

www.pulsetoday.co.uk

www.theconversation.com

www.thecourier.co.uk

www.tht.org.uk

www.uksaysnomore.org

www.who.int

www.yoursexualhealthmatters.org.uk

What is sexual health?

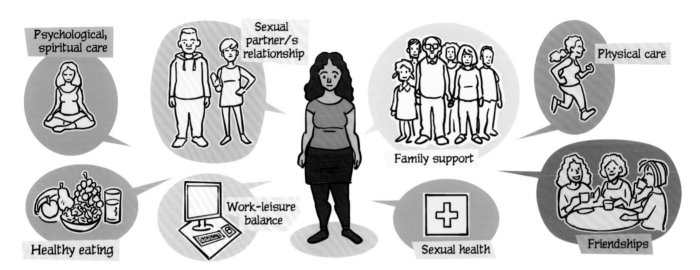

Feeling good

Sexual health is just one part of the bigger health picture. There are lots of components to health – both physical and emotional, and lots of ways that we look after health every day.

Healthy Respect supports the World Health Organisation's idea of sexual health. They say it's not just about steering clear of infections or unwanted pregnancy (though those are important), but also about the right to safe, happy sexual experiences, free from pressure, coercion or harm.

This is the case whether you are male, female or trans, lesbian, gay, bisexual or straight.

So, being sexually healthy is about having safe and respectful relationships, and not having to do anything sexually that you don't want to. Being emotionally OK is a really important part of sexual health too. This means feeling good about your sexual experiences, and not regretting anything that's happened.

Sexuality

Sexuality is unique and different for every individual. It is about all the things that influence how you are as a sexual being, and much more than just your sexual orientation (who you fancy).

Everyone has a right to their sexuality, and to express it (in a safe and legal way). This is true regardless of your age, gender, ability, sexual orientation, religion or beliefs, race or ethnicity, and if you decide to be celibate (not have sex).

Your sexuality is yours and yours alone. It can change over time and can be shaped and influenced by all the following things:

♦ your self image (for example, how you see yourself, your body image, your self-esteem)

♦ your social relationships (for example, family, friends, boyfriends, girlfriends, partners)

♦ your senses (for example, sight, touch, taste, hearing, smell)

♦ your emotions (for example, desire, jealousy, pleasure, anger, intimacy)

♦ your spirituality (for example, beliefs, religion, values, your sense of self)

♦ your political identity (for example, if you have ever faced stigma or discrimination)

♦ your sexual practices (for example, celibacy, sex with a partner, masturbation)

> 'Sexuality is unique and different for every individual.'

Understanding your own sexuality is one way of feeling sexually healthy. This might not always be easy though! If you are ever confused, worried or upset abut your sexuality for any reason, there are places you can go for confidential advice and support.

Physical sexual health

Keeping physically sexually healthy is another aspect of sexual health. This most often means not becoming unwell (e.g. with an STI) or becoming pregnant when you did not want to.

The above information is reprinted with kind permission from *Healthy Respect*.
©2020 HEALTHY RESPECT

www.healthyrespect.co.uk

The changing world of adolescent sexual and reproductive health and rights

The world in which adolescents live has changed dramatically in the last 25 years and the response to their sexual and reproductive health and rights has evolved in important ways.

A new supplement in the Journal of Adolescent Health celebrates gains, confronts barriers, and identifies key areas of action for countries and key stakeholders to build on progress in the critical decade ahead.

The four published articles were developed by technical teams at WHO and UNFPA, along with governments, academia, civil society, and funding organizations. They were co-authored by young people from six regions around the world.

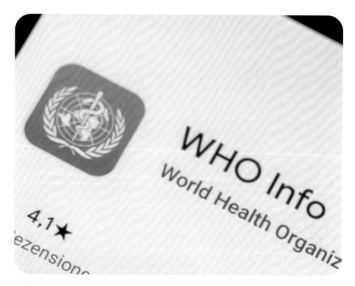

Some positive trends in adolescent sexual and reproductive health and rights

In 1994, the International Conference on Population and Development (ICPD) announced the arrival of adolescent sexuality and adolescent sexual and reproductive health on the global agenda.

An additional 163 million adolescents (aged 10-19) have come of age since then. There are now 1.2 billion adolescents in the world, with diverse interests, needs, and concerns. Many of them are benefiting from shifting development, health, and social trends.

There have been concrete improvements in some aspects of adolescent sexual and reproductive health and rights. Many adolescents initiate sexual activity later than adolescents in the past. They are less likely to have sex with a partner who they are not married to or living with and more likely to use condoms when they are sexually active.

Girls are less likely to be married and to have children before age 18, more likely to use contraception and to obtain maternal health care. They are less likely to experience female genital mutilation, internationally recognised as a human rights violation.

Slow progress for adolescents on other key issues

In spite of greater awareness of the sexual and reproductive health needs of adolescents, some key issues have not improved.

In many contexts, menstruation is still seen as a taboo topic. Adolescents are the only age group in which HIV-related deaths are not decreasing and from the limited data available, their levels of other sexually transmitted infections are high and growing. An unacceptably high proportion of adolescent girls have experienced physical and/or sexual intimate partner violence. There is still a lack of good data on levels of unsafe abortion among adolescents, and the risk of mortality and morbidity resulting from it.

When it comes to gender, adolescents are still expected to conform to specific gender norms. The supplement notes that girls are taught to be 'modest and polite', whereas boys are encouraged to be 'brave and independent'.

These expectations can worsen other inequalities such as those related to poverty, education, and employment, and contribute to differences in adolescent health and well-being along gender lines. For example, while boys are more likely to experience injuries and to use tobacco and alcohol, girls are more likely to experience intimate partner violence.

A time-bound opportunity

Progress over the last 25 years has strengthened the position of adolescent sexual and reproductive health and rights on global, regional, and national agendas. There is more investment and a growing evidence-base, with committed advocacy movements and strong governmental responses in a small but increasing number of countries. This presents new opportunities for all adolescents to achieve and exercise their full potential.

Looking forward, the supplement lays out specific considerations for delivering a comprehensive package of sexual and reproductive health interventions to adolescents. It also proposes specific actions in relation to five strategic areas: political and social support, funding, laws and policies, data and evidence, and the implementation of programmes at scale with quality and equity.

Adolescents have a right to make decisions governing their bodies and to access services that support those rights – and more so than ever before, the international agenda is paying attention.

3 February 2020

The above information is reprinted with kind permission from *World Health Organization*.
©2020 WHO

www.who.int

Fake news: 7 myths about sexual health

Would you consider yourself a sexpert, or does your knowledge about sexual health need a refresh? Misbeliefs around sexual health can have damaging consequences. Better2Know are here to bust the myths and get the facts straight.

There are many misconceptions about sexual health and sexually transmitted infections (STIs). Whether it is something you read online or heard from a friend, false information can be very misleading. It's important to know the facts in order to keep safe and protect your health. So, here are 7 myths – and their truths!

Myth: 'If I had an STI, I would know about it'

Fact: Unfortunately, this is not always the case. Many people with an STI do not show any symptoms of an infection. In fact, around 80% of women and 50% of men do not show any signs of Chlamydia. Regular testing is always advised to make sure an STI does not go undetected.

Myth: 'An STI will eventually disappear without treatment'

Fact: An STI will not go away by itself. However, most STIs can be easily treated and cured with a course of antibiotics. Early detection is important. The longer an infection is left untreated, the more serious the potential health implications become. These health risks vary depending on the type of infection, ranging from infertility, pelvic inflammatory disease (PID) and damage to vital organs in the body.

Myth: 'A swab test is painful and embarrassing'

Fact: You may feel uncomfortable at the idea of having a swab taken, but the process is quick, simple, and pain-free. Our clinicians have seen it all before, so there is no need to feel embarrassed. You are taking responsibility for your sexual health which is the most important thing to remember.

Myth: 'STIs only affect young people who have sex with multiple people'

Fact: As the saying goes, once is enough to catch a sexually transmitted infection. Anyone who is sexually active is at risk of catching an STI – no matter their age, gender, or sexuality. STIs do not discriminate and nobody is immune.

Myth: 'If I use a condom, I am protected against all STIs'

Fact: Apart from abstaining from sex, condoms are the most effective method to prevent STIs. However, they are not 100% effective and do not cover the whole genital area. It is possible to catch some infections including Herpes and Syphilis through skin-on-skin contact alone.

Myth: 'My STI test and results will appear on my medical records forever'

Fact: When you test with Better2Know, all your personal information is kept private and confidential. We will never share your results with anyone else without your permission. If it makes you feel more comfortable, you can even choose to be anonymous for your tests.

Myth: 'You cannot catch Herpes from someone unless they are having an outbreak'

Fact: Herpes can be spread even when a person has no visible symptoms. This is known as a process called 'asymptomatic viral shedding'. It most often happens in the early stages of infection, and just before or after an outbreak.

24 July 2020

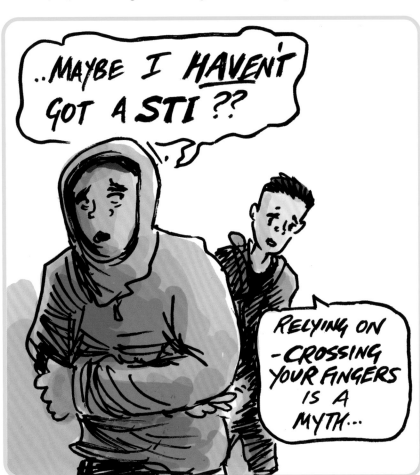

..MAYBE I HAVEN'T GOT A STI ??

RELYING ON -CROSSING YOUR FINGERS IS A MYTH...

The above information is reprinted with kind permission from *Better2Know*. ©2020 Better2Know Limited

www.better2know.co.uk

10 MEGA MYTHS about sex

There are lots of things said about sex that aren't really true.

1. Real life sex is like pornography

Not true: People taking part in most pornography are paid actors and they're doing things to entertain the people watching it.

Often, the things that happen all the time in porn aren't really common in everyday sex, but watching lots of porn can make people believe they are.

The way porn stars look is often very different to real life too.

2. Everyone is having sex

Not true: The decision to have sex is not about what other people are doing. Having sex is a personal choice and just because you have done it before, doesn't mean you have to do it again.

If you don't feel ready, you're not ready. You may not feel ready until you meet someone you trust and are comfortable with, and it's the next step in your relationship at a time that's right for both of you.

3. Boys don't need to worry about contraception, that is the girl's responsibility

Not true: The decision to have sex is a joint one. You might believe your girlfriend is on the pill or taking other contraception, but this is only effective if taken correctly.

Also, the only way to protect against a sexually transmitted infection (STI) is by using a condom.

4. STI tests are only for those who sleep around

Not true: Anyone who has unprotected oral, vaginal and anal sex can catch an STI, so it's always best to practise safe sex.

It's not always possible to tell if someone has an STI, and they might not even realise themselves if they don't have any symptoms.

Yearly tests are recommended, or each time you want to sleep with a different partner.

5. You can't get pregnant if you have sex in a bath, standing up or on your first time

Not true: There are lots of myths around having sex, buts that's exactly what they are – myths!

If you have any unprotected sex at any time, you are at risk of getting pregnant.

6. I would be able to tell if my partner had a STI

Not true: There is no way of being certain that your partner doesn't have an STI unless you both have been tested.

Before you consider having sex, it's important to talk to your partner about a full STI screen to make sure you both know for certain.

Condoms are the best protection for you both against STIs.

7. You can't use condoms if you're allergic to latex

Not true: Condoms come in all different sizes and latex-free condoms are also available if you have a latex allergy.

If you struggle to use condoms, take time to practise putting them on so you feel more comfortable with using them.

8. If he 'pulls out' when he comes (ejaculates), she can't get pregnant

Not true: Before a boy ejaculates, there's sperm in the pre-ejaculatory fluid (sometimes called pre-come), which leaks out when he gets an erection.

It only takes one sperm to get a girl pregnant. If you have unprotected sex, you're at risk of pregnancy and of catching an STI.

9. Drinking alcohol or using drugs aren't good when it comes to sex

True: When you're drunk or under the influence of drugs, it's hard to make smart decisions.

Alcohol and drugs can make you take risks, such as having sex before you're ready, or having sex with someone you don't trust.

You're more likely to regret having sex if you do it when you're drunk. You may also be at risk of a sexual assault and rape. If you're too drunk, you can't legally consent to sex.

10. You have to use emergency contraception the morning after sex

Not true: This is a common misconception due to the nickname for the emergency hormonal contraception pill being the 'morning after pill'.

The emergency contraception pill can be given up to 5 days after unprotected sex, although the sooner it's taken the better.

If you're worried you have missed this time frame, there are other options available, so speak to your school nurse.

The above information is reprinted with kind permission from *Health For Teens*.
©2020

www.healthforteens.co.uk

Who should have the HPV vaccine?

There are 2 human papillomavirus (HPV) vaccination programmes in England. One is for children who are 12 to 13 years of age, and one is for men who have sex with men (MSM) up to 45 years of age.

The universal HPV vaccination programme

In England, all boys and girls aged 12 to 13 years are routinely offered the 1st HPV vaccination when they're in Year 8 at school. The 2nd dose is offered 6 to 24 months after the 1st dose.

If you're eligible and miss the HPV vaccine offered in Year 8 at school, you can get it for free on the NHS up until your 25th birthday. Contact your school immunisation team or GP surgery.

The vaccine is effective at stopping people getting the high-risk types of HPV that cause cancer, including most cervical cancers and some anal, genital, mouth and throat (head and neck) cancers.

It's important to have both doses to be properly protected.

Who should not be vaccinated?

The HPV vaccine should not be given to people who:

♦ have had a severe allergic reaction (anaphylaxis) to a previous dose of the HPV vaccine or any of its ingredients

♦ are known to be pregnant

Who should delay vaccination?

HPV vaccination should be delayed for people who are unwell and have a high temperature, or are feeling hot and shivery.

This is to avoid confusing the symptoms of the illness with the response to the vaccine.

There's no reason to delay vaccination for a mild illness, such as the common cold.

What if you miss your vaccine?

Anyone who misses either of their HPV vaccine doses when they became eligible in school Year 8 should speak to their school immunisation team or their GP surgery. They should make an appointment to get up to date as soon as possible.

If you have the 1st dose of the HPV vaccine at 15 years of age or over, you'll need 3 doses to be fully protected. Having 2 doses is not as effective for older people.

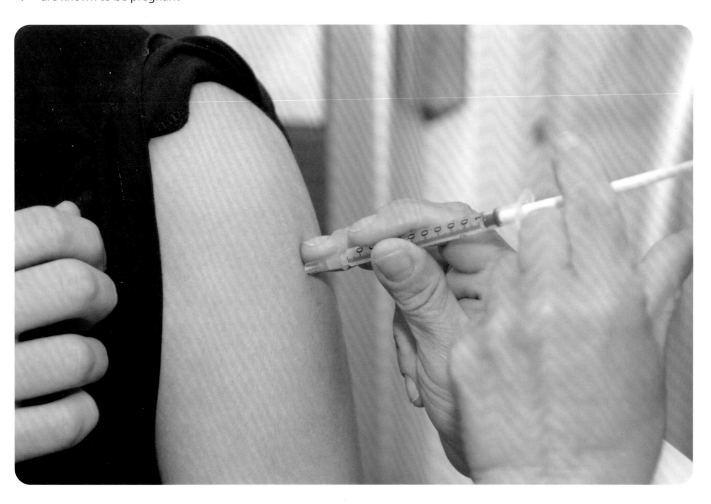

The HPV vaccine and men who have sex with men (MSM)

The longstanding HPV vaccination programme in girls indirectly protects boys against cancers and genital warts linked to infection with HPV because girls will not pass HPV on to them.

MSM have not benefited in the same way from the girls' HPV vaccination programme.

But they're at risk of cancers linked to infection with HPV types 16 and 18 that affect men, such as cancer of the anus, penis, mouth or throat.

MSM are also at risk of genital warts caused by HPV types 6 and 11.

MSM up to and including the age of 45 are eligible for free HPV vaccination on the NHS when they visit sexual health or HIV clinics.

MSM aged 15 and over need 3 doses of the vaccine. Those under 15 need 2. It's important to have all doses to be properly protected.

Ask the doctor or nurse at the clinic for more details.

Transgender people and the HPV vaccine

Some transgender people are also eligible for the HPV vaccine.

Trans women (people who were assigned male at birth) are eligible for the HPV vaccine if their risk of getting HPV is similar to the risk of MSM who are eligible for the HPV vaccine.

Trans men (people who were assigned female at birth) are eligible if they have sex with other men and are aged 45 or under.

If trans men have previously completed a course of HPV vaccination as part of the girls' HPV vaccine programme, no further doses are needed.

Ask the doctor or nurse at the sexual health or HIV clinic for more details.

10 May 2019

The above information is reprinted with kind permission from *NHS*.
©Crown copyright 2020

www.nhs.uk

Puberty is starting earlier for many children – sex education must catch up with this new reality

An article from The Conversation.

THE CONVERSATION

The British government is consulting on a new curriculum for sex and relationship education in English schools. This change provides a timely opportunity to update how, when and what children are taught about puberty.

Astonishingly, the Department for Education (DfE) guidance on sex education has not changed for nearly two decades. But after concerted lobbying, research, and the recommendations of multiple committees of MPs, in 2017, the Children and Social Work Act finally acknowledged the need to provide "sex education for the 21st century".

New statutory guidance for schools will be published following the public consultation, which closes in mid February. From 2019, secondary schools will be obliged to offer relationships and sex education, and primary schools to offer relationships education.

Parents will retain the right to remove their children from sex education – other than that which is covered in the science curriculum – but will not be allowed to remove them from relationships education.

These changes are underpinned by widespread concern about the negative effects of digital technologies on young people's sexual lives, particularly sexting, child sexual abuse and exploitation, and "strangers online". The new curriculum will, it seems, teach children and young people what healthy relationships look like in the fraught context of smart phones, online porn and Instagram.

The new puberty

But the new curriculum should also take account of what is happening to the bodies of young people in the 21st century. Not only do kids seem to be growing up much faster today, many of them are actually starting to develop physically earlier than ever before.

According to many scientists and clinicians, we are living in the era of " the new puberty" in which increasing numbers of girls start to develop sexually at age seven or eight. In the 1960s, only 1% of girls would enter puberty before their ninth birthday. Today, up to 40% of some populations in both rich and poor countries are doing so.

Sexual development is also being stretched out for longer, with many girls starting to grow breasts and pubic hair two to three years before they have their first period. While there is less evidence that boys' development is changing so rapidly, some studies also indicate that earlier entry into puberty's initial stages is becoming more common.

The causes of these changes remain unclear. Many scientists point to the simultaneous increase in childhood obesity, while others study the effects of environmental chemicals, such as Bisphenol A or BPA (which is found in some plastics), on the body.

Other research has explored the effects of social factors, including family structures, experiences of early life trauma and socioeconomic disadvantage. This range of explanations points to how complex a phenomenon puberty is.

The current DfE guidance states that:

All children, including those who develop earlier than the average, need to know about puberty before they experience the onset of physical changes.

But it leaves schools to decide, in consultation with parents, "the appropriate age" to teach children about puberty. In 2017, the Personal, Social and Health Education Association argued that this should be when they're age seven. But talking to seven year-olds about breasts, pubic hair, body odour and genital changes may not be easy for many teachers, or for many parents. Being seven is supposed to be a time of freedom, play and innocence.

Updating sex education

Children who develop early present a challenge both to cultural thinking about sex and to sex education policy. While many parents and young people want updated sex education, this usually comes with the proviso that such education be "age appropriate".

Although very important, this phrase is painfully vague – and it's unclear whether it refers to chronological age, emotional age or stage of physical development.

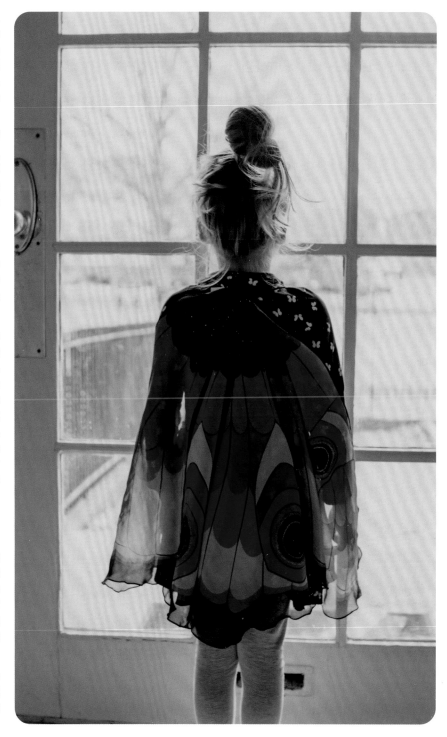

Today, some seven-year-olds may be emotionally young but also starting to grow breasts and pubic hair. Other early developers who have experienced early life stress – such as abandonment or abuse – may feel more mature than their peers and be ready earlier to learn about puberty and sexuality. The widening gap in the timing of boys' and girls' sexual development also poses a challenge. Teaching girls separately, or earlier than boys – the strategy in my own child's primary school – risks reinforcing harmful gender norms and notions of secrecy around issues such as menstruation.

Instead, perhaps we could try to disentangle puberty from teenage sexuality and to develop accounts of puberty that do not frame it as the dawn of adolescence. A seven year-old with breasts is not "becoming a woman", and a menstruating nine-year-old is probably not going to want to have intercourse anytime soon.

Ultimately, this means moving beyond traditional portrayals of female bodies that focus on reproductive capacity in order to explore wider meanings and experiences of being a girl. Growing up is also about new horizons, such as strength, health, even pleasure. Sex and relationships education might even then include puberty as something to be anticipated, noticed, even celebrated – rather than as yet another risk.

18 January 2018

The above information is reprinted with kind permission from The Conversation © 2010-2019, The Conversation Trust (UK) Limited

www.theconversation.com

Women struggling to access usual contraception as coronavirus plunges sexual health services into chaos

'Women are frustrated and annoyed. They don't understand why they can't access the service. They don't want an unwanted pregnancy,' says lead contraceptive nurse.

By Maya Oppenheim, Women's Correspondent

Women are struggling to access their usual methods of contraception due to sexual health services being plunged into chaos in the wake of the coronavirus crisis, service providers have warned.

Sexual health clinics have been shut or are running a skeleton service, as staff have been deployed to other parts of hospitals to help with the coronavirus emergency, while large numbers of GPs are off sick with coronavirus or self-isolating.

A study carried out by the British Association for Sexual Health and HIV since the Covid-19 outbreak found 86 per cent of clinics could not offer the most effective long-acting contraceptive choices of a coil or an implant, and only two-thirds could still fit a coil for emergency contraception.

Tracey Forsyth, lead contraceptive nurse at British Pregnancy Advisory Service, told *The Independent* some sexual health clinics are saying they are open online when they are not.

Ms Forsyth, whose contraceptive team speaks to around 400 women a week via the phone, added: 'GPs are saying "use condoms" to women when they ring up and ask for a repeat prescription of contraceptive pills or ask to have the coil fitted or another form of contraception.

'Women are having difficulty getting access to contraception. They are telling me they can't get long-acting reversible contraception [LARC] fitted at the moment. This includes the implant, coil and injection.

'If someone needs to have an emergency coil that stops them getting pregnant because the condom splits, they should be able to. It is essential contraceptive services are open at this time. Most people I'm speaking to are saying they are having more sex because they have got more time. They may be furloughed and have not got the stress of going out to work.

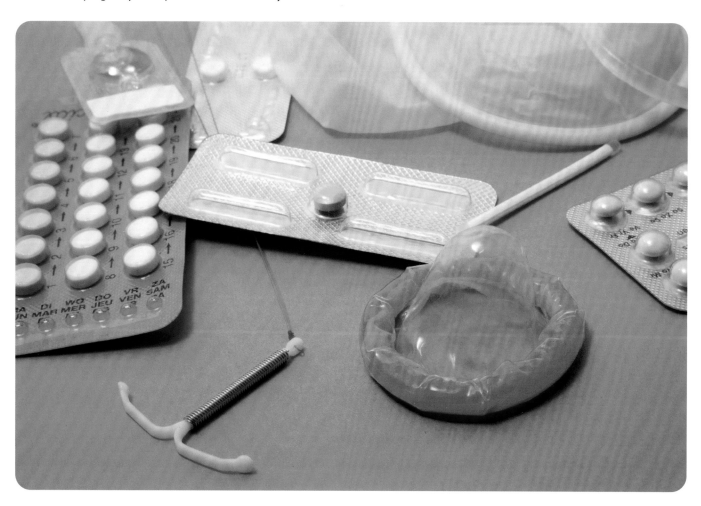

'But women are frustrated and annoyed. They don't understand why they can't access the service. They don't want an unwanted pregnancy. Especially not with the economic uncertainty of the current situation. They are worried about the future and whether they have a job go back to and bills are piling up. Not being able to get contraception is an additional pressure in what is already a difficult situation.'

Ms Forsyth, who has been running the UK-wide contraceptive and sexual health phone service for 11 years, said the Faculty of Sexual and Reproductive Healthcare has released new guidelines in the wake of coronavirus but claimed not all GPs are following them.

The nurse said some GPs are blocking women from getting the contraceptive pill due to not having their blood pressure reading or only having a reading from a year ago, despite the new guidelines stating this is no longer necessary in the wake of the coronavirus crisis.

Ms Forsyth, who said the pandemic was exacerbating existing cuts to sexual health services, noted women she speaks to are fearful of contracting coronavirus while picking up their contraceptive pills from GP clinics. She said some GP practices are only offering a tight time slot to pick up prescriptions, which can be difficult if you are having to juggle collecting them with being at work for set hours.

Peter Greenhouse, spokesperson for the British Association for Sexual Health and HIV, an association of specialists who work in sexual health clinics, said: 'The longer the lockdown goes on, the worse the situation will get for women's sexual health.'

The sexual health consultant, whose organisation carried out a survey of all sexual health clinics in the country, added: 'Anything that limits availability and choice of contraception harms women's health and Covid's had a huge impact on sexual health services. Our UK-wide live survey found that two-thirds of clinics had less than 20 per cent capacity for face-to-face consultations.

'A third of services have stopped giving three-monthly contraceptive injections (Depoprovera), 86 per cent of clinics couldn't offer the most effective long-acting choices of a coil or an implant, and only two-thirds could still fit a coil for emergency contraception.

'Although 90 per cent offer telephone advice on choice and supply of pills, switching methods during the current crisis is more difficult and only one in five clinics can provide pills or patches online. So while social distancing is reducing opportunities for the spread of STIs, women who need to adjust their contraception, or manage heavy or severely painful periods, will have a much more challenging time.'

Anne Lashford, vice president of the Faculty of Sexual and Reproductive Healthcare, said the progestogen-only pill is being prescribed as a 'temporary bridging method' for women who are not able to get a hold of other methods of contraception.

Dr Lashford added: 'For some people, the progesterone pill might not be their ideal form of contraception but they can move back to their preferred method once services are open. You can't predict what sort of bleeding pattern you will get on the progesterone pill. Around half of the women

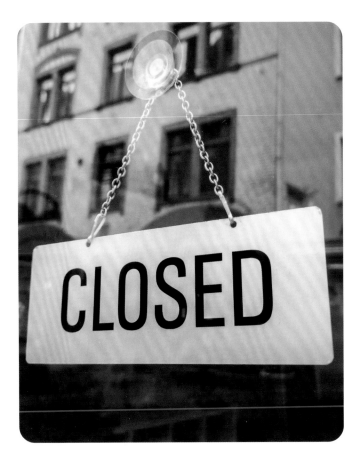

who take it have no periods. Some will have a reasonably regular cycle. Others will have erratic bleeding.

'One group running into some problems is those who have contraceptive injections which need to be done in person every 12 weeks but you can extend to 14 weeks.'

The Faculty of Sexual and Reproductive Healthcare has released new guidance for decision-makers and doctors on how services should be run in the wake of the pandemic – as well as releasing a leaflet with information for women on what contraception they are able to access.

The organisation, which said consultations are now being carried out via phone or video, said the new guidelines advise women to extend the use of their implants or IUDs.

Sexual health services were overstretched before the coronavirus emergency; frontline service providers previously told *The Independent* women's health is being put at risk and abortion rates are rising, because clinics providing women with contraception are being forced to close due to 'damaging' cuts.

Figures show spending on contraception has fallen by almost a fifth since 2015 – with data provided by the Advisory Group on Contraception showing the proportion of councils reducing the number of places providing contraceptive services has risen from just nine per cent in 2015-16 to 26 per cent in 2018-19.

19 April 2020

The above information is reprinted with kind permission from *The Independent*.
© independent.co.uk 2020

www.independent.co.uk

New laws have not stopped women and girls being exiled during their periods in Nepal

An article from The Conversation.

By Melanie Channon, Fran Amery, Jennifer Thomson

THE CONVERSATION

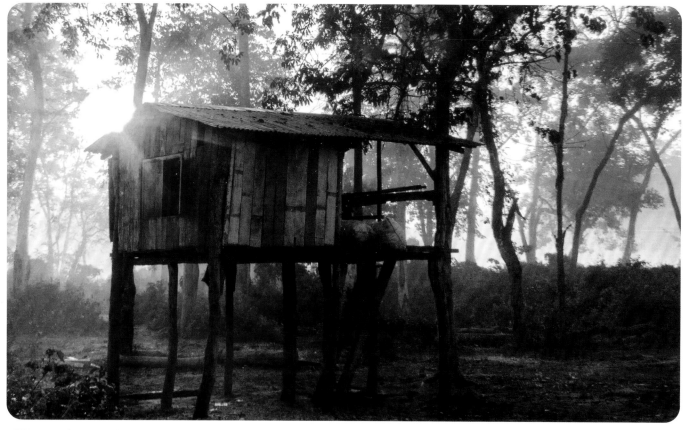

Periods are still treated as a taboo subject in many parts of the world. Despite being a completely normal biological function, they are often seen as shameful, embarrassing and impure.

As a result, a wide variety of customs have developed around menstruation. In Nepal, the breadth and depth of menstrual taboos is particularly severe.

A woman or girl having their period might not be able to sleep in her own bed, engage in religious activities, eat or drink normal food, enter the kitchen, touch (or even look at) other people (especially men), use the family toilet, or even enter the family home.

In the west of the country, a practice known as "chhaupadi" prevails, which means that during menstruation you must sleep outside the family home, traditionally in a purpose built menstrual hut, known as a "chhau goth". Or it might mean sleeping in a communal space above animal sheds, inside those sheds with animals, or even outside in the open air.

This practice has resulted in several deaths, most recently in December 2019, when Parwati Budha Rawat from Achham was so cold she lit a fire and died of suffocation due to lack of ventilation.

Chhaupadi was only officially criminalised in Nepal in August 2018, and enforcing the practice is now punishable by a fine or three months in jail. But the first arrest only occurred last week, in relation to the death in Achham.

And with the woman dead, who will be prepared to speak up? Herein lies the problem with criminalising chhaupadi – it requires women and girls to go to the police and speak out against their own families or neighbours. It would not be possible to report anonymously, so unless the community as a whole decides to outlaw the practice, criminalising it is of little practical use.

In our recent study looking at menstrual practices in the Dailekh district of Nepal (next to Achham district), we found that 77% of girls practised chhaupadi (as did 72% in a separate study of Achham).

We also found that while 60% of girls knew chhaupadi was illegal, knowing about the law made no difference to whether or not it took place. Among those who knew about the law, many felt that it was pointless and couldn't see how it would change anything.

We were told that volunteers had visited villages, informing people about the new chhaupadi law. But girls from those villages said the volunteers were still following chhauppadi in their own homes.

The adolescent girls we spoke to also described the fear and anxiety that came with menstrual taboos. Several said that they wished they had been born boys. One said:

'Some girls are even scared that they might get raped and killed while staying outside. We hear news where girls die due to snakebites while sleeping outside their homes during their menstrual period.'

And while chhaupadi has been criminalised, it is important to remember the many other harmful practices surrounding menstruation across Nepal. These include dietary restrictions, being prevented from going to important social events such as weddings, or simply being seen as unclean and impure. All take their toll on physical and mental health.

So what can be done about such deep-rooted cultural practices? In another part of Nepal, one community leader has responded to the death in Achham by reportedly offering cash to women who reject chhaupadi.

A communal problem

Perhaps a monetary incentive or having a community leader prepared to take a stand will make a difference. The main response to criminalisation so far has been to destroy chhau huts. But this is not helpful, as most women and girls simply sleep in a different (and often less safe) place, frequently with animals or outside.

In our study, 96% of the girls we spoke to were keen to see a change in menstrual restrictions, but they were unsure about how to bring about that change. A lot of campaigns in the past have focused on knowledge about periods, distributing sanitary pads, and maintaining healthy practices.

These have been effective in some ways but do little to address chhaupadi. The girls we spoke to generally already understood menstruation and practised good menstrual hygiene.

We also found that the various cultural practices surrounding menstruation were affecting their mental (as well as physical) health. Despite being well educated about periods, girls did not feel able to fight taboos when so many senior people in their family, the community, and their religion believed in them.

Girls wanted to see change from the top with community and religious leaders taking a stand and publicly discarding practices of "untouchability" and chhaupadi. The government and the law were also discussed, with some saying that they wanted criminalisation strictly enforced, but others saying that this would cause problems if attitudes were not changed.

It is unsurprising that the law is not taken seriously as a force for change when the first arrest took 16 months. Ultimately, change must come from inside communities and cannot be forced by outsiders from Kathmandu or international organisations.

12 December 2019

The above information is reprinted with kind permission from The Conversation
© 2010-2019, The Conversation Trust (UK) Limited

www.theconversation.com

Family planning/ contraception methods

Key facts

♦ Among the 1.9 billion women of reproductive age group (15-49 years) worldwide in 2019, 1.1 billion have a need for family planning; of these, 842 million are using contraceptive methods, and 270 million have an unmet need for contraception [1,2]

♦ The proportion of the need for family planning satisfied by modern methods, Sustainable Development Goals (SDG) indicator 3.7.1, was 75.7% globally in 2019, yet less than half of the need for family planning was met in Middle and Western Africa [1]

♦ Only one contraceptive method, condoms, can prevent both a pregnancy and the transmission of sexually transmitted infections, including HIV.

♦ Use of contraception advances the human right of people to determine the number and spacing of their children.

Brief overview

Ensuring access for all people to their preferred contraceptive methods advances several human rights including the right to life and liberty, freedom of opinion and expression and the right to work and education, as well as bringing significant health and other benefits. Use of contraception prevents pregnancy-related health risks for women, especially for adolescent girls, and when births are separated by less than two years, the infant mortality rate is 45% higher than it is when births are 2-3 years apart and 60% higher than it is when births are four or more years apart[1]. It offers a range of potential non-health benefits that encompass expanded education opportunities and empowerment for women, and sustainable population growth and economic development for countries.

Modern contraceptive prevalence among married women of reproductive age (MWRA) increased worldwide between 2000 and 2019 by 2.1 percentage points from 55.0% (95% UI

53.7%–56.3%) to 57.1% (95% UI 54.6%–59.5%) [1]. Reasons for this slow increase include: limited choice of methods; limited access to services, particularly among young, poorer and unmarried people; fear or experience of side- effects; cultural or religious opposition; poor quality of available services; users' and providers' bias against some methods; and gender-based barriers to accessing services.

Contraceptive methods

Methods of contraception include oral contraceptive pills, implants, injectables, patches, vaginal rings, Intra uterine devices, condoms, male and female sterilization, lactational amenorrhea methods, withdrawal and fertility awareness based methods.

These methods have different mechanisms of action and effectiveness in preventing unintended pregnancy. Effectiveness of methods is measured by the number of pregnancies per 100 women using the method per year. Methods are classified by their effectiveness as commonly used into: Very effective (0–0.9 pregnancies per 100 women); Effective (1-9 pregnancies per 100 women); Moderately effective (10-19 pregnancies per 100 women); Less effective (20 or more pregnancies per 100 women).

22 June 2020

[1] Kantorová V, Wheldon MC, Ueffing P, Dasgupta ANZ (2020) Estimating progress towards meeting women's contraceptive needs in 185 countries: A Bayesian hierarchical modelling study. PLoS Med 17(2):e1003026. https://journals.plos.org/plosmedicine/article?id=10.1371/journal.pmed.1003026

[2] United Nations, Department of Economic and Social Affairs, Population Division. Family Planning and the 2030 Agenda for Sustainable Development. New York: United Nations. https://www.un.org/en/development/desa/population/publications/pdf/family/familyPlanning_DataBooklet_2019.pdf

[3] Family Planning Can Reduce High Infant Mortality Levels. Guttmacher Institute. https://www.guttmacher.org/sites/default/files/report_pdf/ib_2-02.pdf

The above information is reprinted with kind permission from *World Health Organization.* ©2020 WHO

www.who.int

Mechanisms of action and effectiveness of contraceptive methods

Method	How it works	Effectiveness: pregnancies per 100 women per year with consistent and correct use	Effectiveness: pregnancies per 100 women per year as commonly used
Combined oral contraceptives (COCs) or 'the pill'	Prevents the release of eggs from the ovaries (ovulation)	0.3	7
Progestogen-only pills (POPs) or "the minipill"	Thickens cervical mucous to block sperm and egg from meeting and prevents ovulation	0.3	7
Implants	Thickens cervical mucous to block sperm and egg from meeting and prevents ovulation	0.1	0.1
Progestogen-only injectables	Thickens cervical mucous to block sperm and egg from meeting and prevents ovulation	0.2	4
Monthly injectables or combined injectable contraceptives (CIC)	Prevents the release of eggs from the ovaries (ovulation)	0.05	3
Combined contraceptive patch and combined contraceptive vaginal ring (CVR)	Prevents the release of eggs from the ovaries (ovulation)	0.3 (for patch) 0.3 (for CVR)	7 (for patch) 7 (for CVR)

Intrauterine device (IUD): copper containing	Copper component damages sperm and prevents it from meeting the egg	0.6	0.8
Intrauterine device (IUD) levonorgestrel	Thickens cervical mucous to block sperm and egg from meeting	0.5	0.7
Male condoms	Forms a barrier to prevent sperm and egg from meeting	2	13
Female condoms	Forms a barrier to prevent sperm and egg from meeting	5	21
Male sterilization (Vasectomy)	Keeps sperm out of ejaculated semen	0.1	0.15
Female sterilization (tubal ligation)	Eggs are blocked from meeting sperm	0.5	0.5
Lactational amenorrhea method (LAM)	Prevents the release of eggs from the ovaries (ovulation)	0.9 (in six months)	2 (in six months)
Standard Days Method or SDM	Prevents pregnancy by avoiding unprotected vaginal sex during most fertile days.	5	12
Basal Body Temperature (BBT) Method	Prevents pregnancy by avoiding unprotected vaginal sex during most fertile days.	Reliable effectiveness rates are not available	
TwoDay method	Prevents pregnancy by avoiding unprotected vaginal sex during most fertile days.	4	14
Sympto-thermal method	Prevents pregnancy by avoiding unprotected vaginal sex during most fertile days.	<1	2
Emergency contraception pills (ulipristal acetate 30 mgor levonorgestrel 1.5 mg)	Prevents or delays the release of eggs from the ovaries. Pills taken to prevent pregnancy up to 5 days after unprotected sex	<1 for ulipristal acetate ECPs, 1 for progestin-only ECPs, 2 for combined estrogen and progestin ECPs	
Calendar method or rhythm method	The couple prevents pregnancy by avoiding unprotected vaginal sex during the 1st and last estimated fertile days, by abstaining or using a condom.	Reliable effectiveness rates are not avaialble	15
Withdrawal (coitus interruptus)	Tries to keep sperm out of the woman's body, preventing fertilization	4	20

Collapse in sexual health checks after funding cuts driving soaring STI rates, Labour suggests

Syphilis, gonorrhoea and chlamydia all on the rise.

By Colin Drury

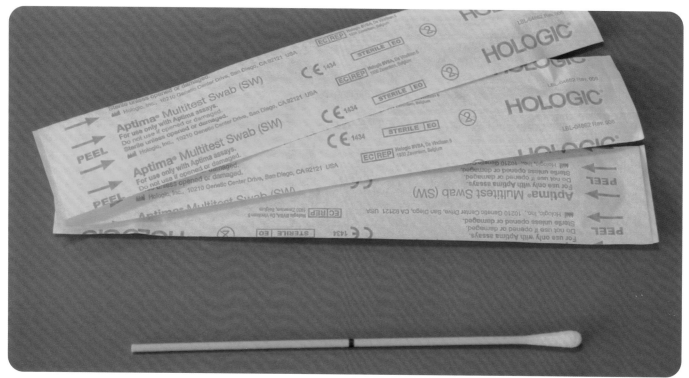

Sexually transmitted infections are soaring across England as new figures show the number of people receiving sexual health checks has collapsed as budgets have been cut.

STIs such as syphilis, gonorrhoea and chlamydia are all on the rise, Public Health England has previously warned.

Now, health minister Steve Brine has admitted that related health checks have fallen by 245,000 in the past three years.

He disclosed the figure in parliament after House of Commons library figures were found to reveal the sexual health budgets of local councils had been slashed by £55.7m since 2013/14.

Shadow health secretary Jon Ashworth said: "These deep cuts are completely shortsighted and will only lead to wider pressures on the NHS in the long term.

"The government can't be taken seriously on its commitment to prevention while at the same time cutting vital services that provide contraception, tackle sexually transmitted infections and offer crucial support and advice."

He added that Labour would now use an opposition day motion in parliament to try and force the government to reverse cuts to public health budgets.

Mr Ashworth said: "I will demand that ministers start by reversing these swingeing cuts to public health provision and publish their equality impact assessments so we can see the effects these cuts are having on society."

A Department of Health and Social Care spokesperson said the decision on how money was spent on local public health services rested with individual authorities themselves.

He said: "We have a strong track record on sexual health with teenage pregnancies at an all-time low and sexually transmitted infections continuing to fall. Sexual health services and tests are now more widely available online – more than 11,000 diagnoses from online tests were reported last year."

Public Health England's most recent figures show some 422,000 STIs were diagnosed in England in 2017, up from 415,000 a decade earlier.

12 May 2019

The above information is reprinted with kind permission from *The Independent*.
© independent.co.uk 2020

www.independent.co.uk

New STI stats show action urgently needed to tackle soaring rates

Today's figures published by Public Health England show there were 447,694 sexually transmitted infections (STIs) reported in England in 2018.

Gonorrhoea cases are up 26% on the year before and the highest number in over 40 years, with syphilis up 5% from 2017.

The key statistics are:

◆ 249% rise in gonorrhoea from 2009 and 26% from 2017.

◆ 165% increase in syphilis from 2009 and an increase of 5% from 2017.

◆ 22% drop in chlamydia testing of young people (15-24 years) since 2014.

◆ Overall STI rates up by 5% on the year before, when there were 422,147 new STI diagnoses.

◆ Attendance at sexual health services has risen 15% in five years.

Debbie Laycock, Head of Policy and Public Affairs at Terrence Higgins Trust, said:

'Today's new STI statistics shows there needs to be urgent action to improve the state of the nation's sexual health. We are yet again seeing soaring rates of syphilis and gonorrhoea, and increases in the number of people attending sexual health services, which is happening against a backdrop of central government stripping £700m from public health budgets in the last five years.

'The Government cannot bury its head any longer – the consequences of under investment and services struggling to meet demand is plain to see with these STI numbers.

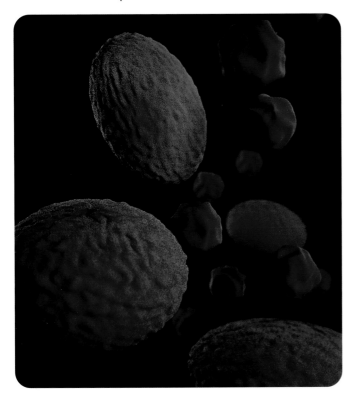

'Progress has sharply halted in tackling rates of chlamydia, with rates up 6% last year while there continues to be a decline in the number of chlamydia tests being carried out. This is clear evidence that removing access to testing is having a direct impact on the rates of chlamydia, with cases now rising.'

The data shows that certain groups are disproportionately affected by STIs. On this, Debbie Laycock added:

'The impact of continued slashing of sexual health budgets was laid bare in a report by the Health Select Committee just two days ago. It revealed there is now a real risk to widening health inequalities already faced by certain groups.

'These groups – including BAME communities, young people, people living with HIV and gay and bisexual men – are once again disproportionately affected by new STI rates. Gay and bisexual men for example accounted for 75% of new syphilis cases.

'A range of sexual health services must be available, including different options for testing and support, but this must not come at the expense of vital face-to-face services.

'We welcome the long-overdue decision to include BAME-specific data in today's report, which has revealed large variation in STI diagnoses between ethnic groups. This is an important step in understanding the sexual health needs and experiences of different communities. However, this must be translated into targeted interventions to support people to access sexual health services.

'Going forward, lessons must be learned from sexual health interventions that have seen positive results. The continued fall in new HIV diagnoses has seen the Government commit to ending new transmissions by 2030, while the introduction of the HPV vaccine to girls – which is due to be extended to boys this year – has resulted in rates of genital warts declining. We urgently need that same decisive action to get a grip of other rising STIs.

'That's why we are calling on the Government to show leadership by urgently committing to an ambitious national sexual health strategy which fast-tracks action to address STIs. Sexual health funding must be increased as part of the forthcoming spending review to ensure services can properly meet local demand.

'Today's STI statistics, combined with the serious warning from MPs, demonstrates very clearly the dire impact on sexual health that decisions being made by central Government are having. Ministers need to wake up to this crisis and take decisive action. Their handling of sexual health to date is simply not good enough.'

4 June 2019

The above information is reprinted with kind permission from Terrence Higgins Trust.
©2020 Terrence Higgins Trust

www.tht.org.uk

New approaches needed to care for youth with HIV

Youth make up a growing share of those with HIV and are less likely to medicate properly. New approaches are needed to protect youth.

By Natasha Comeau

Young people, who represent a growing share of those with the AIDS virus, are struggling to follow the prescribed course of medication to control HIV, and new approaches are needed to help them suppress the infection.

A person with the human immunodeficiency virus (HIV) used to be doomed to die, but that is no longer the case. By taking a daily pill, someone with HIV can lead a long and healthy life, and not contract acquired immunodeficiency syndrome (AIDS).

But that means taking antiretroviral medication. A recent study of HIV care for young adults that tracked newly-diagnosed U.S. youth found only 12% of participants achieved viral suppression after five months.

Viral suppression is crucial for both "the health of the self and the health of others," said one of the study's authors, Kenneth Mayer, professor of medicine at Harvard Medical School. Viral suppression reduces HIV to undetectable levels and prevents transmission of the virus to others.

Of the 1,411 newly diagnosed HIV-positive youth who participated in the study published in the Journal of Acquired Immune Deficiency Syndrome (JAIDS), one quarter failed to access care at all and only 166, or 12%, achieved viral suppression. That compares to an overall viral suppression rate of 60% in the U.S. population.

Addressing the treatment gap is crucial. Globally, more than 30% of all new HIV infections occur in young people aged 15 to 25, according to the World Health Organization (WHO). And a growing number of children are infected with HIV at birth.

Today, more than five million young people live with HIV, according to the WHO.

Care barriers

"Treating HIV can be really daunting for young people because antiretroviral medication is a lifelong commitment," said Alexis Palmer-Fluevog, Health Science professor at Langara College in Vancouver, Canada. Daily medication is currently the only way to maintain viral suppression, and the virus can rebound very quickly.

Youth face a host of barriers that make it harder for them to obtain treatment and to remain on antiretrovirals.

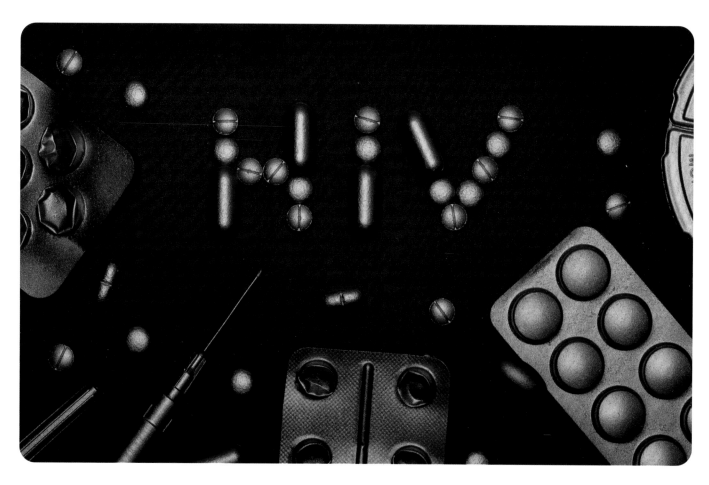

"For some individuals, there are simply economic barriers," Mayer said. In Canada, antiretrovirals cost around US$10,600, a year according to the Ontario Ministry of Health. In the United States, the cost is US$39,000, according to Medicaid data.

Apathy can be a problem

Prices elsewhere vary considerably. Medication in Switzerland and Germany costs more than €20,000 a year, according to the European Centre for Disease Prevention and Control (ECDC). But 91% and 84% of these costs, respectively, are covered by health insurance.

Meanwhile, in some counties with much lower antiretroviral prices, like Latvia and Lithuania, less than 30% of the costs are covered, according to the ECDC.

Awareness can be an issue. "Almost half of youth who are HIV-infected in the U.S. are unaware of their status," Mayer said. By comparison, 85% of those older people infected with HIV in the United States know their status, a study on the HIV continuum of care has found.

Apathy can pose problems. Many people are less concerned about dying from HIV than they once were.

"This is what we call 'therapeutic optimism,'" Mayer said. "HIV is not the lethal disease it once was in the '80s." Treatment is better than ever before, and there is pre-exposure prophylaxis, or PrEP, which offers people at risk daily medicine to lower their chances of getting the HIV virus, according to the U.S. Centers for Disease Control and Prevention (CDC).

Compounded vulnerability

Youth who have the hardest time suppressing the virus include the homeless, those with significant behavioral or mental health issues, those with substance-abuse problems and survivors of trauma.

For these HIV-positive youth, treatment may compete with other priorities, such as finding housing or treating addiction.

There is also mistrust in the healthcare system, which can limit engagement and care for some individuals, especially those from communities of colour, which have long suffered racism in the HIV/AIDS epidemic that continues today.

"People of colour report being disrespected, experiencing microaggressions and other kinds of anticipatory problems in seeking care," Mayer said, referring to individuals who will not seek care if they anticipate discrimination or racism.

What is more, HIV can be associated with homophobia, dissuading some people from seeking care. "The population where HIV is least controlled in the United States is among young men of colour who have sex with other men," Mayer said.

"There are high levels of perceived and experienced stigma around HIV, particularly for youth growing up in non-affirming environments," Mayer said. These youth may not be comfortable seeking care because they do not want others to know their status and are concerned about their privacy.

Targeted solutions

Better health interventions are needed to combat the spread of HIV among young people. "Currently, there is a real lack of youth-friendly messaging and services," said Palmer-Fluevog.

Education is a starting point. Condom use has declined, people tend to have more sexual partners than in the past and many HIV-positive youth do not know they are infected, according to the CDC. These issues could be addressed with safe sex education, better public health information about the risks of HIV transmission and incentives to complete sexual health checkups.

Rapid testing and treatment are crucial. "The shorter the time between a positive HIV test result and being brought to a clinic for treatment, the more likely they will have longer term viral suppression," said Bill Kapogiannis, the lead author of the JAIDS study and a physician at Eunice Kennedy Shriver National Institute of Child Health and Human Development.

The "gamification" of HIV treatment

It is essential to develop strategies to ensure HIV-positive youth remain in care. Of the youth tracked in the JAIDS study, barely one third remained in care after five months.

"Gamification" of HIV treatment could help youth take their medication, research from the Desmond Tutu HIV Foundation in Cape Town, South Africa has shown. For example, pill-taking could be turned into a game played on a smartphone. A number of such apps have been developed, but they remain in clinical trials.

South Africa offers adherence clubs, where people with HIV can pick up pills and discuss treatment issues with other HIV patients. The clubs ensure adherence to treatment at much higher rates than traditional clinics.

6 April 2020

QUESTIONS TO CONSIDER:

♦   1. When it comes to fighting AIDS, why is viral suppression so important?

♦   2. Why do HIV-positive youth have greater difficulty suppressing the virus than the general population?

♦   3. Which of the targeted solutions in the article do you think are most likely to be successful and why?

Natasha Comeau is a fellow in global journalism at the Dalla Lana School of Public Health at the University of Toronto. She holds a Masters of Global Affairs from the Munk School at the University of Toronto, where she focused her studies on development and global health. Comeau has also written for News Decoder on at-home testing for STDs and youth inactivity levels.

The above information is reprinted with kind permission from News Decoder.
© News Decoder 2020

www.news-decoder.com

HIV diagnoses at lowest level since 2000 thanks to testing and prevention efforts

By Anviksha Patel

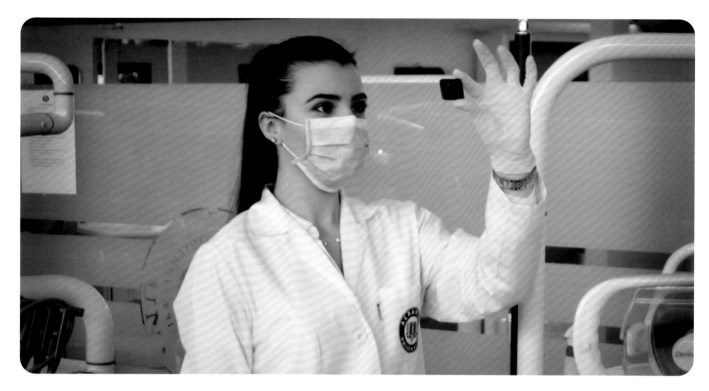

The number of new HIV diagnoses in the UK has fallen by almost a third since 2015 and is at its lowest level since 2000, figures by Public Health England have revealed.

Data has shown there were 4,484 new diagnoses of HIV in 2018 compared to 6,271 in 2015 – a decline of 28%.

PHE said this was due to 'enormous' testing and prevention efforts in the UK.

Diagnoses have fallen in both gay and bisexual and heterosexual populations, according to PHE data. However, the steepest falls are among gay and bisexual men where there has been a 39% decline since 2015.

Within that group, the biggest decline has been among gay and bisexual men living in London and those between 15 and 24, with diagnoses decreasing by 50% and 47% respectively.

Between 2015 and 2018, new HIV diagnoses amongst heterosexual populations fell by 24%.

However, PHE has said the challenge in early diagnosis remains. Over 40% of new diagnoses in 2018 were at a late stage of infection, which increases the risk of death within one year by ten-fold.

The decline has been put down to HIV prevention policies over the last decade, including HIV testing, condom provision, the increased use of pre-exposure prophylaxis (PrEP) and anti-retroviral therapy (ART) drugs that maintain the low level of HIV in the body and prevents the virus from being passed on.

PHE head of HIV surveillance Dr Valerie Delpech said: 'It is thanks to the enormous testing and prevention efforts in the UK that we are seeing further declines in new HIV diagnoses, which have now reached their lowest in almost 20 years.'

She added: 'Getting tested for HIV has never been easier, with free tests available through GP surgeries, local hospitals and sexual health clinics, as well as through a self-sampling service or by using a self-testing kit. Early diagnosis means early effective treatment, which can prevent you passing on HIV.'

Public health minister Jo Churchill said: 'This decline in diagnoses is a result of our unwavering commitment to prevention which has led to more people getting tested and has allowed people with HIV to benefit from effective treatment, stopping the virus from spreading further. 'However, I am not complacent and remain dedicated to ensuring we reach our target of zero new HIV transmissions by 2030.'

It comes as researchers suggested GPs need more than one-off training sessions to encourage them to offer more HIV tests.

11 September 2019

The above information is reprinted with kind permission from *PULSE*.
© Cogora 2020

www.pulsetoday.co.uk

As STIs in older people continue to rise Age UK calls to end the stigma about sex and intimacy in later life

To address and challenge the negative stereotypes of sex and intimacy in later life Age UK, working in partnership with a Manchester based coalition, is running a social media campaign highlighting that older people are diverse in their desire for sexual intimacy and that anyone of any age can get sexually transmitted infections.

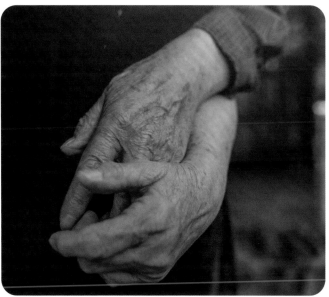

The campaign, which started on Monday 30 September, is running for 5 days and is centred around International Older People's Day, on Tuesday 1 October. It has been developed by a Manchester based coalition of academic, public and voluntary sector organisations called the Sexual Health of Older People (SHOP) working group.

The campaign is tackling themes around sexual safety and the need to use protection at any age, access to health services and how these need to be appropriate for people of all ages, as well as tackling issues such as diversity, women's health and emotional intimacy.

In 2018 there were nearly three times more new diagnoses of sexually transmitted infections (STIs) among men aged 45-64 than among women in the same age group.

Men in this age group received 23,943 diagnoses of STIs, an 18% increase since 2014, while women received 8,837 diagnoses, a 4% increase since 2014.

Between 2014 and 2018 there was a reduction in the rate of new STI diagnoses in men aged 20-24 (7.3% less than in 2014) whereas in men aged 45-64 there was a 13.9% increase. There was also a 23% increase in diagnoses amongst both men and women aged 65+ between 2014 and 2018.

These figures show that STIs are a significant problem among older people and that there are increasing inequalities in sexual health between older and younger men, and between older men and older women.

Sex in later life can be seen as embarrassing and unmentionable but sexual relationships provide physical, mental and emotional health benefits for people, regardless of age. The achievement of sexual wellbeing can play an important part in older people's relationships and being comfortable talking about sex is essential to avoiding STIs.

In fact, analysis of the English Longitudinal Study of Ageing (ELSA) shows that 80% of people aged 75+ agree that satisfactory sexual relations are essential to the maintenance of a long-term relationship. However, many people may not be getting the support from health care professionals that they need to remain sexually active as they get older.

Caroline Abrahams, Age UK's Charity Director, said: "Sex continues to be important for many of us well into old age, but for some reason the whole topic remains taboo in some circles. This is a shame and it also means that sexually active older people are at greater risk of STIs than they need to be or ought to be. Health professionals should be open about discussing sexual health with older people and certainly not immediately jump to the conclusion that sex is irrelevant once you pass a certain birthday. Public health messages around sexual health and STI prevention also need to recognise the reality that sex is a part of many people's later lives and aim to be inclusive of people of all ages."

Dr Dave Lee, Reader in Epidemiology and Gerontology at Manchester Metropolitan University says, "The sexual health of older people should not be overlooked by health care professionals in the broader context of maintaining well-being during ageing.

"Recognising that sexual health may be an unspoken quality of life issue for older individuals could also improve the relationship between physician and patients, with better outcomes for the latter."

The social media campaign material also includes taglines suggested by older Mancunians, who attended an engagement and consultation workshop we held on Valentine's Day this year. This campaign is one strand of working being taken forward by the SHOP working group as part of Manchester's WHO Age Friendly City initiative.

Councillor Mary Watson, Lead Member for Ageing, Manchester City Council said, "Manchester City Council works hard to address the negative images and portrayal of ageing that older people tell us negatively impact on their confidence, self-esteem and wellbeing. This year, to celebrate International Day of Older People, we want to work together to be 'age proud' about intimacy in later life."

7 October 2019

The above information is reprinted with kind permission from Age UK.
© Age UK Group and/or its National Partners (Age NI, Age Scotland and Age Cymru) 2020

www.ageuk.org.uk

Preventing STIs

What is the scale of the problem?

STIs are a major public health concern, which may seriously impact the health and wellbeing of affected individuals, as well as being costly to healthcare services. If left undiagnosed and untreated, common STIs can cause a range of complications and long-term health problems, from adverse pregnancy outcomes to neonatal and infant infections, and cardiovascular and neurological damage.

In 2018, there were 447,694 new diagnoses of STIs made at sexual health services (SHSs) in England, a 5% increase since 2017 when 422,147 new STI diagnoses were made. Of these, the most commonly diagnosed STIs were:

♦   chlamydia (49% of all new diagnoses)

♦   first episode genital warts (13%)

♦   gonorrhoea (13%)

♦   first episode genital herpes (8%)

Gonorrhoea and syphilis have re-emerged as major public health concerns, especially among gay, bisexual and other men who have sex with men (MSM). In 2018, 47% of gonorrhoea and 75% of syphilis diagnoses were in MSM. Since 2009, gonorrhoea and syphilis diagnoses have risen by 249% and 165%, respectively overall, and by 643% and 236% among MSM. Higher risk behavioural changes, including more condomless sex with new or casual partners, likely contribute to these trends.

The diagnosis rates of STIs remains greatest in young heterosexuals aged 15 to 24 years, black minority ethnic (BME) populations, MSM, and people residing in the most deprived areas in England.

Preventing common STIs

This edition of Health Matters focuses specifically on the prevention of common STIs, as prevention is central to achieving good sexual health outcomes.

Prime responsibility for prevention rests with local authorities, who commission and support a range of work, often working collaboratively with PHE and the NHS.

The prevention work covered in this edition include:

♦   open access to SHSs, in person or online

♦   relationships and sex education (RSE)

♦   PHE's national HIV Prevention and Sexual Health Promotion programme

♦   the National Chlamydia Screening Programme (NCSP)

♦   the National HPV Immunisation Programme

♦   the Syphilis Action Plan

For example, the National HPV Immunisation Programme is a preventative measure as it delivers the HPV vaccine, which protects against 4 types of HPV. These include both high- and low-risk types responsible for the majority of cervical cancers and genital warts. By 2058, the programme could prevent up to 64,138 HPV-related cervical cancers and almost 50,000 other HPV-related cancers.

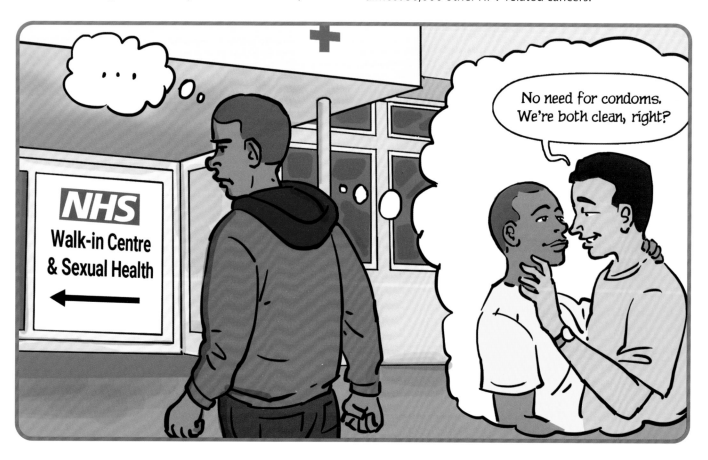

Funding and commissioning sexual health services

Responsibility for commissioning sexual health, reproductive health and HIV serivices is shared across local authorities, clinical commissioning groups and NHS England.

Local authorities

- Comprehensive sexual health services including most contraceptive services and all prescribing costs, but excluding GP additionally-provided contraception

- STI testing and treatment, chlamydia screening and HIV testing

- Specialist services, including young people's sexual health, teenage pregnancy services, outreach, HIV prevention sexual health promotion, services in school, colleges and pharmacies.

Clinical commissioning groups

- Most abortion services

- Sterilisation

- Vasectomy

- Non-sexual-health elements of psychosexual health services

- Gynaecology including any use of contraception for non-contraceptive purposes.

NHS England

- Contraception provided as an additional service under GP contract

- HIV treatment and care (including drugs costs for PEPSE)

- Promotion of opportunistic testing and treatment for STIs and patient-requested testing by GPs

- Sexual health elements of prison health services

- Sexual assault referral centres

- Cervical screening

- Specialist fetal medicine services

Antimicrobial resistance in STIs

Increasing resistance and decreasing susceptibility to antimicrobials used to treat STIs has reduced treatment options, and are therefore emerging concerns.

This is particularly the case for gonorrhoea, as there are no classes of antimicrobials to which gonorrhoea has not developed resistance. As a result of this, first-line gonorrhoea treatment in the UK was recently changed from dual therapy of ceftriaxone with azithromycin, to monotherapy with ceftriaxone at a higher dose.

Fortunately, ceftriaxone resistance remains rare in the UK. However, in 2018, there were 3 cases of extensively drug-resistant gonorrhoea detected in the UK, which included ceftriaxone resistance.

With patterns of antimicrobial resistance (AMR) having the potential to change rapidly, ongoing monitoring of AMR is vital to ensure that first-line treatment remains effective. Ineffective treatment facilitates onward transmission and adverse sequelae.

Collaboratively commissioning SHSs

Responsibility for commissioning sexual health, reproductive health and HIV services is shared across local authorities, clinical commissioning groups (CCGs) and NHS England. These shared responsibilities require a whole system approach to commissioning of these services. PHE and others have published a range of guidance to support this approach, which you can find in the full edition online.

The recently published Prevention Green Paper outlines that government would like to see the NHS and local authorities working more closely at both the national and local level to make collaborative commission the norm, building on best practice from across the country.

It also sets out that the shift towards Integrated Care Systems (ICSs) creates the opportunity to co-commission an integrated sexual and reproductive health service.

There are different ways of taking collaborative commissioning forward and each local area should decide what suits them best, using their existing powers and levers to develop joint approaches.

Call to action

The full edition suggests several calls to action for preventing STIs, including:

- preparing for the implementation of relationships education and RSE at primary and secondary level, respectively

- using condom distribution schemes

- using data, evidence and PHE's resources including health economics tools to support decisions around commissioning SHSs

- commissioning collaboratively and whole-system working between commissioners

- delivering testing and treatment using existing frameworks and pathways, such as the chlamydia care pathway

- managing local STI outbreak and incidents with the support of PHE's national guidance and national reference laboratory

21 August 2019

The above information is reprinted with kind permission from Public Health England.
©2020 Crown copyright

www.publichealthmatters.blog.gov.uk

What are the chances of getting an STI?

The chances of getting an STI are probably lower than you think, but here's why having safer sex is still a very good idea.

By Justin Hancock

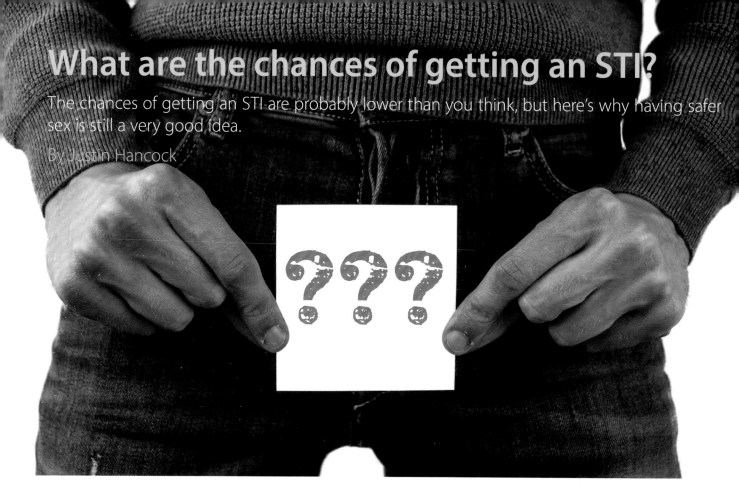

Whenever we see statistics in the news about STIs they are often using the actual numbers of cases, because these actual numbers look quite big. People want to make the numbers look big because:

♦ it makes a juicy scary news story blaming all these 'naughty irresponsible people over there' for not wrapping up;

♦ or, less commonly, to make a point about the dreadful under-funding of sexual health services and outreach services;

♦ or, even less commonly, to make a point about how drug companies need to be investing more in drugs to treat/cure these infections but they won't because there isn't a great deal of profit in making new antibiotics.

Annnnnyway, so they make the numbers look big. Public Health England reported that 144,000 young people, in England, were diagnosed with Chlamydia or Gonorrhoea in 2017. That is a lot of people: too many people. However, it's probably not as many as you think when you realise that there are 6,935,586 young people in England. So even though I did my GCSE in Maths in 1991 I reckon that means that around 2% of young people have Chlamydia or Gonorrhoea. Other studies suggest that the actual rate of Chlamydia in young people might be around 3% (ie, not just those that have been diagnosed).

Gonorrhoea is much less common than Chlamydia, with 11,261 young people being diagnosed with it in 2017. So that's more like 0.16% of young people living in England – which is still too many young people, but it's not an epidemic. There were 278 cases of Syphilis among young people.

If the chances of getting an STI are so low, why bother with safer sex?

Obviously, if everyone decided to stop using condoms, getting tested, or having safer sex then these numbers would go up. One reason that we should try to have safer sex is that we are taking part in a social practice to reduce social harms. Just like sneezing into a tissue or covering our mouth when we cough. It's good and nice to take care of ourselves and other people, so let's keep trying to do that if we can.

Our chances of getting an STI vary enormously and it's kinda random.

Also our chances of getting an STI vary enormously and it's kinda random. We can only get a sexually transmitted infection by having unprotected sex with someone who has a sexually transmitted infection. That person would have got their STI from someone else they had sex with, that person would have got their STI from someone they had sex with etc etc. Because a lot of people have sex with someone that they live near (particularly young people), and young people are more likely to change partners, then outbreaks of STIs are often very local.

Where there are outbreaks over a bigger geographical area, for example in a big city, then it's because people travel to have sex. So it might not be geographically local, but they will be part of an IRL social network of people who are shagging each other. Often we either know other people that other people are shagging, or we know of them — one or two cases of an STI in one of these groups makes the chances of getting an infection a lot higher. It won't affect a huge number of people in a city, but in that social network of people it will.

So although there might be a 0.16% chance of getting Gonorrhoea in England, the truth is that in some areas it will be 0% chance (because no-one has it) and in other areas it might be more like 5-10%, because loads of people, who might have sex with each other, have it. So it could be your estate, your village, your workplace, your community, your college, your Uni, that club that everyone goes to, that holiday resort…. We don't really go about saying 'yeah this Uni has a Gonorrhoea problem', but if a sexual health service shows up and gives you condoms and information about where your local services are then you should probably listen.

Why is it important?

Well I think it's important to give factual, correct information – call me old fashioned – and to base our decisions on that. As I've explained above, we don't always know what our actual risks of getting an STI are so it's important not to be complacent about safer sex.

As I've explained in this blog and about chances of getting pregnant, if people are taught that their risks are way higher than they actually are then it can have a counter productive effect. This is what happens:

♦ people have unprotected sex a few times;

♦ think 'nothing bad has happened, I must be infertile/immune to STIs*',

♦ so they don't get into the habit of safer sex; and then they get an STI, or have an unplanned pregnancy. (*that's not how STIs work btw)

The other thing that panicking about STIs does is to put people off going to sexual health services. Making STIs seem a lot worse and a lot more common than they are creates a stigma that puts people off going to clinics. I've written more about that at my blog for sex educators (please stop showing pictures of infected genitals thanks). Because many STIs don't have symptoms, the only way that we might find out that we have an infection is by having a check up. Not getting tested means that we might be infecting other people, creating our own social network of risk. If we also have an STI without getting treatment then we might run the risk of getting serious infections. So getting tested is super important.

So let's have an appropriate level of concern about how common STIs are. I'm not saying chill and don't bother using condoms/having safer sex. I'm saying let's make our decisions about how to look after our sexual health based on all the facts.

5 November 2019

For more RSE teaching resources for practitioners visit bishtraining.com

The above information is reprinted with kind permission from *Justin Hancock*.
© 2020 Bish UK

www.bishuk.com

Getting tested for STIs

Sexually transmitted infections (STIs) are any kind of bacterial or viral infection that can be passed on through unprotected sexual contact. They can have a number of signs and symptoms, however, some STIs have no symptoms, and if left untreated can lead to infertility.

If you are worried that you might have a STI, you can get free advice and testing from Brook clinics, sexual health services (or GUM clinics), young people's services, your GP or free online STI kits.

Contraception and sexual health services such as Brook are free and confidential, including for people under the age of 16. Health professionals work to strict guidelines and won't tell anyone else about your visit unless they believe you're at serious risk of immediate harm. Find out more about Brook's confidentiality policy.

What will an STI test involve?

First of all, the doctor or nurse will discuss with you what tests they think you will need and these tests will probably depend on how you answer some questions about your medical and sexual health.

These questions will include:

♦ when you last had sex

♦ whether you've had any unprotected sex

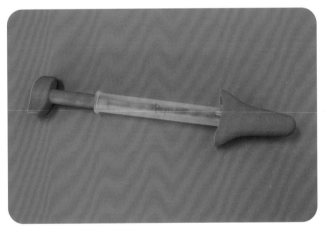

♦ whether you have any symptoms

It is recommended that you answer these questions as honestly as possible so you can get the help and advice you need. And there's no need to be embarrassed! The people who work in sexual health clinics have seen and heard it all. Trust us!

The STI tests might involve:

♦ Giving a urine (wee) sample

♦ Giving a blood sample

♦ Taking swabs from the urethra (the tube urine comes out of)

♦ Swabs from the vagina (you can often take these yourself)

♦ An examination of (a look at) your genitals

These tests and examinations are nothing to worry about and the doctor or nurse will help you to feel comfortable.

Here's a bit more about each type of test

Swabs

The swab looks like a small cotton bud which is wiped over the vagina or from the tip of the penis. Very often you can take the swab from inside the vagina yourself. If you have had oral or anal sex then a swab may also be taken from either your throat or rectum. Taking the swab may be slightly uncomfortable but should not be painful.

Urine tests

A urine sample involves weeing into a small pot which your doctor or nurse will give you. You can collect the urine sample at any time of day (unless you are advised otherwise) and you will also be told if the sample needs to be the first part of the urine sample or a 'mid stream' sample. You will also need to wash your hands before and after taking the urine sample.

Blood tests

A sample of blood is taken from your arm and sent off to a laboratory to be tested. You are usually sitting down and a tight band called a tourniquet is put around your upper arm to make it easier to take the sample of blood. They will ensure that the skin is clean and a needle attached to a syringe will be inserted into the vein. This isn't usually painful and you may feel a slight pricking sensation as the needle goes in. If you are worried or feel faint tell the health professional as they can help to make you feel more comfortable. After the needle has been removed they will apply pressure for a few minutes and a plaster/cotton wool pad will be left on. Some services can also test for some STIs via a finger prick blood test which can give results on the same day.

How is each STI tested?

When you visit the clinic you will discuss which tests you will require with the doctor or nurse. Here is an overview of which tests are commonly used to diagnose each type of STI:

♦ Chlamydia: tests usually involve giving a urine sample or taking a swab

♦ Gonorrhoea: tests usually involve taking a swab or giving a urine sample

♦ Genital herpes: the doctor or nurse may be able to diagnose genital herpes by

looking at the affected area – however, taking a swab of fluid from a blister will confirm this

♦ HIV: the most common way of testing for HIV involves taking a small sample of blood. HIV can be detected in the body four weeks after exposure to the virus

♦ Syphilis: diagnosis usually involves an examination, followed by swabs (if there are sores) and a blood test. The blood test is usually repeated after three months

♦ Pubic lice: diagnosis involves a health professional examining the area with a magnifying glass

♦ Trichomoniasis: tested for by taking a swab or urine sample

♦ Genital warts: diagnosis involves a health professional examining the area

How long will I wait for results?

Some sexual health services can do a test which produces the results during the appointment time (this is called 'point of care testing'). Or they make take a swab and then look at the sample under a microscope in order to diagnose it during your visit.

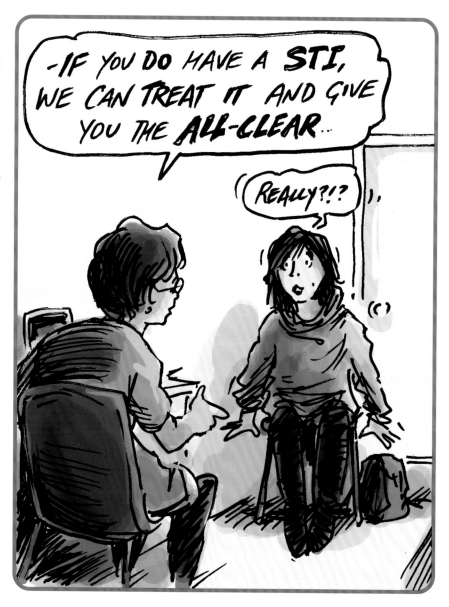

Otherwise the swab may be sent away to a lab, in which case the results normally take a week to come back.

If you have your STI test done at Brook we will let you know how you will receive your results at your appointment.

What happens if my test shows I've got an STI?

Most STIs can be easily treated with antibiotics. If you test positive for any STI, your clinic will encourage you to talk to your current partner and sometimes to your previous partners so they can be tested as well. The clinic will help you find the best way to talk to other people if you need to, and can notify, even contact them for you through 'partner notification' and not even mention your name.

STIs can be treated as below:

- Chlamydia: is treated with a course of antibiotics. The two most commonly prescribed treatments are: Azithromycin (single dose) or Doxycycline (a longer course, usually two capsules a day for a week)

- Gonorrhoea: treatment usually involves having an antibiotic injection and a single dose of antibiotic tablets

- Genital herpes: treated with antiviral medicines (although there is no cure)

- HIV: HIV is preventable (through using condoms) and treatable (with drugs called antiretrovirals), but it is not curable

- Syphilis: usually treated with a single antibiotic injection or a course of injections

- Pubic lice: treatment can be done at home using special types of insecticide lotions, creams or shampoo

- Trichomoniasis: treated with antibiotics, usually a five to seven day course of an antibiotic called Metronidazole

- Genital warts: treatment will depend on how many you have but may involve creams or freezing (cryotherapy)

- Most antibiotics are safe to use with hormonal contraception (like the pill, patch, injection or implant) but talk to the person prescribing the treatment to make sure

- Tell the nurse or doctor if you are pregnant or think you may be, or if you are breastfeeding. This will affect the type of antibiotic you are given

- Side effects of antibiotics are usually very mild but may include stomach ache, diarrhoea, feeling sick and thrush

DON'T PASS IT ON

You should also avoid having sex until you have been given the all-clear, to prevent you being re-infected or passing the infection on.

I'm really nervous about going!

Don't be! It's really common to feel nervous at the thought of getting tested; however to reassure you, most infections are easily treated.

For many people, whether it's your first time or not, visiting a sexual health clinic can cause a bit of anxiety. It may ease your worry if you know that:

- They've seen it all. Clinic staff see all kinds of things. After all, it's their job. Staff are there to make your visit as comfortable as possible.

- It's confidential. This means they won't tell your parents, teachers or anyone else unless they think you are at risk of immediate harm. Read more about confidentiality.

- You can be seen soon. Many clinics have walk-in hours where you can just show up and be seen. It's a good idea to call to see if you need an appointment and if the clinic offers drop-in appointments, expect to wait a while when you get there.

What will happen when I get there?

When you go to get an STI test you can either make an appointment or attend a drop-in service. For some drop-in services you may need to wait while.

At the clinic you will be asked your name and contact details – your GP will not be told about your visit unless you have given your permission, and your visit will be confidential unless they think you are at serious risk of immediate harm.

During your consultation the doctor or nurse will ask you some questions about your sexual history including when you last had sex and whether you have had unprotected sex. They will then talk you through the test.

You will be asked how you would like to receive your results, this can be via phone, text message or unmarked post. Depending on the type of test you have, some results are available straight away and you may be given treatment to take away with you on the day, but others will need to be sent away to a laboratory and you will usually be contacted in one-two weeks.

If you test positive for an STI you will be asked to come back to the clinic to talk to discuss treatment. The clinic can also notify your previous sexual partners through 'partner notification' if you don't feel comfortable doing this yourself.

14 August 2019

The above information is reprinted with kind permission from Brook.
©2020 Brook Young People

www.brook.org.uk

Guide to relationships

By Justin Hancock

In this guide to relationship we'll learn about: what we mean by relationships; limits; how you should be treated; romance; trust; and break ups.

What did you learn about relationships at school or at home? Not a lot I bet. I think most of us learn about relationships from doing them. From seeing other people and their relationships and also from discussing relationships with each other.

Short version

Learn from one kind of relationship, like a friend, to help you with another, like a bae. Consent and limits are really important. To try to be clear and honest about what you want and what you can give. Don't try to neg people into giving you what you want. You should feel part of a team, like someone who is your best friend.

It's actually okay to argue so long as you don't try to hurt each other. Be careful about doing everything with just one person. Remember that you have a relationship with yourself. Lastly remember that there are often good reasons why relationships should end. We see being in a relationship as being better than single, well it's not. It's certainly better to be single than be in a bad relationship.

That's the summary, read on for that deep dive content.

What are relationships?

Lots of people worry about the word 'relationship' because it sounds heavy. Hook ups, FWBs, seeing each other, dating, going out, boy/girlfriend, engaged, partnered, married are all relationships, just different types. Going even further than that: friends, family, classmates, teammates, colleagues are all relationships too. How we feel about ourselves is also a relationship: I mean, even having a pet is a relationship.

The point is that there is a lot in common with all different kinds of relationships. So you could learn about what works for you in one relationship when you are having problems with another one. If you're going out with someone who puts you down all the time you could ask yourself 'if this was

a mate, would that be okay?' They are just different kinds of relationships and there is more than one kind of love. Thinking about your own relationships this way then you can make your own guide to relationships to work out what works for you.

Limits

Pressuring or forcing your partner to go beyond their sexual limits is VERY BAD. As is pressuring or forcing someone into being a parent, or get married, or to say they love you. If someone is pressuring you into going beyond your limits then you could maybe dump them.

Consent is just as important in relationships as it is in sex. So as well as setting limits and respecting other people's limits, you should try to make it consensual where there aren't clear limits. For example, give people options about what they would like to do. Make this more than just an option of 'shall we do this or not do this'. Also keep paying attention to how the other person is feeling and check in with them to make sure. There are lots of reasons why people find it hard to state what their limits are in relationships.

Treat 'em mean, they should dump you

You've heard the expression, 'treat 'em mean, keep 'em keen'? WRONG! Dating and relationships aren't a battle, or a 'game'. Other guides to relationships are like that, but they are wrong. Be like a really good mate. Encourage rather than make them feel small. Be generous with your time and resources. Support them. Work together as a team. You should expect to feel this in return too.

However, it is also possible to be a bit much sometimes. Some people like someone to be there for them a lot, others like a bit of distance. That doesn't mean that you should just play it cool all the time just in case, but it does mean that you should probably have a conversation about it. It can be hard chatting about relationships (and I've got that advice about how you can talk about talking).

Argue, but do it properly

Arguments can be well upsetting, particularly if you are in a new relationship and haven't had one before. It can be scary because it might make you think that the relationship isn't meant to be. This means that people often try to avoid arguments but that is a bad idea. Being able to say that you are unhappy with someone, and to be able to hear that they are unhappy with you, is an important part of relationships. Relationships can improve hugely after an argument (and why people feel closer afterwards). So long as you both really listen to each other and agree a course of action afterwards.

So good arguing isn't about winning and losing, it's about communicating. About what's wrong and what's upsetting you and listening to what your partner is saying to you. This is easier said than done. There's a difference between having an argument and a row (a yell, not a row as in rowing a boat). Rowing can be an important way of telling people that you are pissed off and that they should take you seriously. However, it's hard to be clear when you are rowing and it's really hard to listen to other people (which is an essential bit).

So try to notice your feelings when you are in the middle of an argument and own them. If you notice that you are angry then you should just say to yourself, 'I'm angry'. The other person can then tell you what their feelings are and you can then talk about how you are going to do this. For example, it might be a good idea to have a time out so that you can calm down. This is especially a good idea if anger is in danger of turning into aggression. Then you can talk about how you are going to have the argument (rather than have a row).

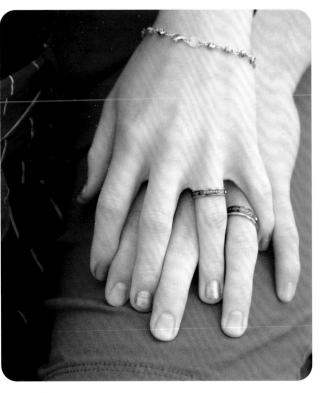

One way to do this is to spend 5 minutes listening to your partner, giving them enough time and space to clarify what it is that is annoying them, then summarise what they just said to prove you were listening. Then change around so the other gets their say. That way stuff gets sorted. You could also try having a text exchange, or putting it all in a google doc and getting them to respond (which is very trendy and really works). If things are super difficult you could try and find someone who could be a go between: someone who knows you both equally and who can step in and help you communicate. If you do this you should really do something nice for them afterwards, because that is a hard job.

Romance

So not everyone likes doing romance or even romantic relationships (just like there are asexual folk there are also aromantic folk). If you really want to do romantic relationships and do romantic things then that can be nice.

However, it's important to be consensual and be romantic with someone rather than at someone. Some people like big romantic gestures, some people like surprises, some people really really don't like either. So, again, try to talk about what kind of romance you might both be up for.

You don't need loads of cash to do lovely romantic things. Long walks, picnics in the park, random museum trips, joint selfies, swapping jumpers so you smell each other when they aren't around, making them playlists (or mixtapes if you are 43) and cards, candle-lit KFC (shout out to Morley's though). I've got a few more ideas for how to be romantic on a budget (which I pull out whenever it's Valentine's Day).

However, being romantic is also about just being there with them, giving people your undivided attention. Not looking at your phone all the time. Being able to be vulnerable with someone. Looking into someone's eyes for ages and feeling all tingly and smiley.

If one person really wants all of this romantic stuff and the other just wants to shag, it might be a sign you aren't on the same page. However, being romantic and sexual are not the same thing anyway. Some people want sexual relationships without romance, some people want romantic relationships without sex. We can also have super romantic times with our mates – and sometimes we should put mates before dates. You might also want to think about why people have romantic relationships and think about what you want from them too.

There's a 'U' in couple

Make sure you still spend time doing you and also tending to your other relationships. I think all relationships need a bit of distance for them to work but how much of this is up to you. Some people like to feel close and part of a double act: you know those couples who are always referred to jointly rather than separately. That can feel nice, but other people can feel like that's too much.

It's often a sign of a bad or unhealthy relationship if one person isn't happy about the other person having their own friends, their own interests and their own plans for their future.

It's important to stick to your own game plan about what you have planned for your future. This is because a) relationships often end and b) it makes your relationship stronger if you grow as individuals too. If you're in a relationship and the other person is very controlling and doesn't let you have any life outside of the relationship then it might be a good time to think about whether it is an abusive relationship or not.

Be fair

Everyone has their own ideas about what's acceptable in a relationship, but I think it's important to be fair to each other. It's a good idea to talk about this so that you both know what to expect from each other. For instance, is it ok to see other people? If so, is there a limit on this? Is this fair for both people? (Like, if it's ok for one person to have other sex or romantic relationships can the other?)

Also make your own rules together about how decisions are made in the relationship that affect you. Eg "Why did you say we were going out on Saturday without asking me first?" This all comes back to consent again. Don't assume that someone is up for a thing because they've done it before. Give people lots of options. Give people an out from doing a thing if you feel like they don't want to.

Trust

Lots of people think that trust is the most important element of a good relationship, but what does trust mean?

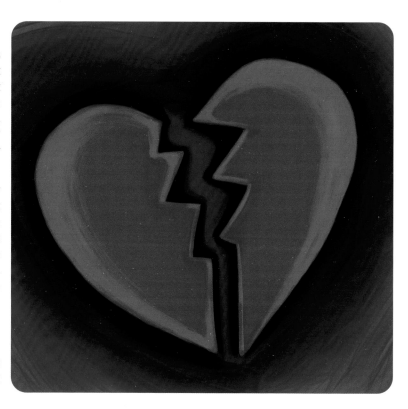

For some people this means 100% honesty. Other people think other things are more important, like: can you trust that they aren't going to hurt you? Can you trust that they would do the right thing about safer sex? Do you believe what they say? Are you able to be fair, and listen to each other, and try to care for each other? If you both follow the advice on here then you might build trust with each other, but it's up to you to figure out when you can trust someone. How do you do know?

If someone has had difficult times in relationships with other people in the past then it may be difficult for them to trust other people. If you're in a situation of you trusting someone more than they can trust you then you may have to be a little more patient. However, if you're in a situation of finding trusting people very difficult then you might have to think about what kind of relationship might actually be right for you right now.

Break ups

*** spoiler***

All relationships end, either through someone dying or a break up. Even if you follow this guide to relationships, it will end.

sorry

However a relationship ends it's important to remember that they can suck for both of you. I think that it's good to be as good and nice as you can about a break-up. For more about this visit my post about breaking up. If you are sure that the relationship has to end: be clear, be honest and avoid giving mixed messages.

Okay so this sounds weird, but I think that it might be a good idea to talk about how you might want to break up. Like, do you want to have these conversations in person or via text? Do you need someone else to intervene and help you

break up (who might be able to help collect stuff or relay messages)? How do you tell people about it? Are you going to follow each other on social media? Do you want to have contact or do you want to have a break for a bit? It's likely that the reason you're breaking up is that you can't have these conversations, so that might not work.

The best break ups are when people can recognise that their relationship can't give them what they need and they both agree. Sometimes these kinds of break ups feel more like a change in the relationship rather than an ending. In those cases it might be that it changes to a different kind of relationship: like going from a romantic relationship to a friendship. That can still be really difficult to do, and it's not cool to just be 'let's be friends' if you're not going to be friends. Perhaps you could be more honest and say 'I don't know how things are going to be between us, so let's see how we feel.' Or 'I can't promise to be friends because we're both changing and growing all the time and I don't know.'

But if your partner was dangerous, nasty, controlling, deliberately made you feel like total shit or was generally awful: be as bad and as loud as you like and just get out. If you don't know how you will ever get over them, I've got that advice for you too.

If you're a teacher or a sex educator, thanks for reading but why not check out my teaching resources like Love, Innit that are designed for you. There are also free RSE resources which I worked on at DO…. These will help young people to make their own guide to relationships.

6 July 2020

For more RSE teaching resources for practitioners visit bishtraining.com

The above information is reprinted with kind permission from *Justin Hancock.*
© 2020 Bish UK

www.bishuk.com

What is relationship abuse?

Abuse in relationships can happen to anyone. It's not normal, it's never OK and definitely not part of a healthy relationship. It isn't always physical, it can be emotional and sexual abuse too. If your relationship leaves you feeling scared, intimidated or controlled, it's possible you're in an abusive relationship.

Is there ever an excuse for relationship abuse?

No there's never an excuse for relationship abuse. Anger, jealousy, alcohol or wanting to protect the other person – none of these are excuses.

How to spot relationship abuse

Some people think that relationship abuse is just about violence, or physically forcing somebody to do something they don't want to – but that isn't true. Abuse can be emotional and verbal, and could escalate to physical or sexual abuse. All types are serious and they're never OK.

What is emotional abuse?

Some people use emotional abuse to control people. These signs can be more difficult to spot, but could include:

♦ Getting angry when you want to spend time with your friends

♦ Isolating you from friends and family

♦ Threatening to spread rumours about you

♦ Saying things like "If you loved me you would…"

♦ Putting you down all the time, using names like 'frigid' or 'slut' to control what you do, humiliate you and destroy your self-esteem

♦ Trying to control your life (telling you how to dress, who you hang out with and what you say)

♦ Threatening to harm you or to self–harm if you leave them

♦ Demanding to know where you are all the time

♦ Monitoring your calls and emails, threatening you if you don't respond instantly

♦ Getting really angry, really quickly

♦ Using force during an argument

♦ Blaming others for their problems or feelings

♦ Being verbally abusive

♦ Using threatening behaviour towards others

♦ Pressuring you to send them nude pictures

If someone is lesbian, gay, bi or transgender and not 'out', their partner might threaten to 'out' them if they don't do what they want.

What is physical abuse?

Some people use violence to force someone to do something or threaten to use it to control them. It could include:

♦ Hitting

♦ Punching

♦ Kicking

♦ Slapping

♦ Pushing someone against a wall and refusing to let them go

♦ Holding somebody down

What is sexual abuse?

Forcing someone to do any sexual acts they don't want to is rape or sexual assault. This kind of abuse can happen in relationships.

Effects and consequences of relationship abuse

Relationship abuse and controlling behaviour can have serious consequences for both the people being abused and those that are doing something wrong to their partners.

How can relationship abuse affect the person being abused?

Relationship abuse can destroy someone's self-confidence, have a negative impact on their health and wellbeing and leave them feeling isolated, lonely or depressed.

What happens to the abusers?

Many abusive behaviours are illegal and can even carry a prison sentence. Criminal convictions can also stop people from doing certain jobs, and travelling abroad to certain countries. So it could seriously damage their future ambitions.

The social consequences of being labelled an abuser should not be underestimated and can be severe. It can have an effect on what people think about you and whether you can get a boyfriend or girlfriend. Would you want to be friends with somebody that was known as an abuser? Now imagine if that person were you.

Advice on relationship abuse

An abusive relationship isn't normal, it's not OK, and if it's happening to you, you're not to blame for the abuse. It might feel like you're alone, but you're not – you deserve to be safe and help is available.

It is important to seek help, but if you're experiencing abuse, you shouldn't confront your abuser on your own. Instead speak to a trusted adult (family member, teacher, youth worker or the police) about what's happening to you.

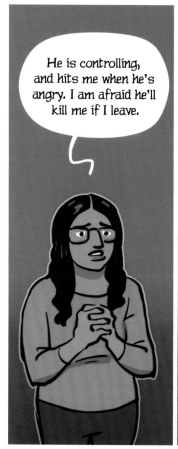
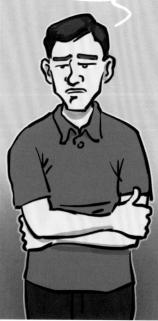
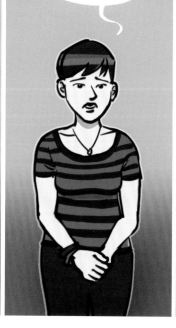
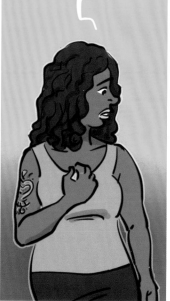

If someone you know is in an abusive relationship, you shouldn't confront the abuser on your own either, but you can seek help on their behalf in a way that is safe for you and them.

You can speak to someone in confidence about abuse in relationships and how to get help – whatever your sexuality or gender identity. You can also speak to the police.

If you, or someone you know, is ever in immediate danger, call 999.

What if you're a boy being abused by a girl?

If you're a young man who's experiencing abuse from your female partner then it may be especially hard for you to tell someone. Some people have told us they would feel less manly if someone knew they were being abused by a girl, or if their female partner threatened them with false allegations in order to keep them silent.

Talk to an adult you trust, it's really important, or speak in confidence to the helplines specifically for men.

What if you're lesbian, gay, bi-sexual or transgender (LGB or T)?

If you're lesbian, gay, bisexual or transgender, you can speak to organisations with people who understand what you are going through. You can also contact the Galop National LGBT Domestic Abuse helpline run by trained advisors.

I'm worried about a friend, what should I do?

It can be really worrying when someone you care about is being hurt or abused by their partner. The more supported your friend feels, the easier it could be for them to deal with what's happening. It's hard to understand when you're not in that situation, so listen, don't be critical and don't pressure them to do something they're not ready to do.

I think I might be abusive, what should I do?

If you recognise the signs of an abusive relationship, and you're hurting the one you love, it can be tough facing up to this, but you can stop and change your behaviour. Call the Respect phoneline – 0808 8024040 – who are experts in talking to people who are abusing their partners.

Are you in a gang and worried about abuse?

Sometimes young people in gangs feel they don't have choices and have to do what's expected of them from other gang members, be it sexual or illegal.

If you're in a gang and you're being pressured or expected to engage in any activity you don't want to do, seek help,. Contact Childline – 0800 1111– to speak to a trained advisor who understands the pressures of being involved in a gang.

The above information is reprinted with kind permission from DISRESPECT NOBODY.
© 2020 Crown copyright

www.disrespectnobody.co.uk

What is consent?

Consent means giving permission for something to happen or agreeing to do something and being comfortable with that decision. It doesn't matter what gender you are, or whether you're straight, gay or bisexual, if you're planning to do anything sexual then both of you must give consent.

Consent has to be given freely and no one can be made to consent to something. It's not consent if someone does something because they feel like they have to. You can also never assume that someone is giving consent – you have to be sure.

Consent is an essential part of healthy relationships and it's really important to know what it is and the many ways to spot it. Both you and the person you're with always need to consent before sex or any intimate activity.

If you want to do something sexual with your partner, the responsibility lies with you to check for consent, not with your partner to say 'no' if they don't want to.

Recognising consent

Consent is an essential part of a healthy relationship, as it's crucial to respect the other person's wishes. It's important to know how to recognise consent because you need to have it for everything sexual that you do together.

You need to take responsibility for seeking consent from your partner every time, as people can change their mind at any point, even during sex. Just because someone consented to something once, it still means you have to ask again as they could feel differently from last time. Also, consent to one sort of sexual activity does not mean consent to everything.

Talk to the other person and check if they're happy.

Good communication is a really important part of a healthy relationship.

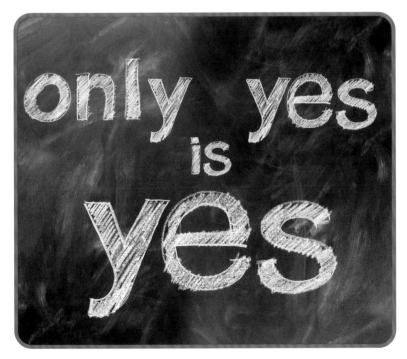

Body language

They may tell you verbally that they do or do not consent to sex or they may show you through their body language. Someone cannot assume another person is giving consent. Remember they don't have to actually say the word 'no' and that they can communicate through body language just as much as speech.

If your partner seems tense, they may be nervous or frightened and are probably trying to hide how they feel.

They may stop kissing you, or not want to be touched or hugged.

These could be signs of non-consent, so don't ignore them – check with the other person.

Being pressured to give consent

If somebody agrees to sexual activity because they've been pestered, intimidated, or faced physical or emotional threats, they have not given consent. Consent needs to be given freely.

Signs of being pressured to give consent can include:

- Being made to feel stupid or bad for saying 'no'
- Being made to feel you have to
- Someone might try to pressure you by calling you frigid or say 'if you loved me you would . . .'
- Being encouraged to drink lots of alcohol or take drugs to make you more likely to have sex
- Making someone feel bad for changing their mind
- Someone might try to pressure you into something to 'prove' you are not lesbian, gay, bi, or transgender

Someone has to have capacity to give consent – what does this mean?

People have to be able to freely give their consent. So if someone's unconscious, drunk or asleep, they cannot freely give consent. Someone may have consented to sex whilst awake, but if they then pass out or fall asleep before you're finished, you have to stop. You can't assume they want to carry on.

Consequences of not giving or getting consent

Pressuring someone to give consent

Pressuring someone into sex is either 'rape' or 'sexual assault', depending on who is involved and what happens. The consequences of both rape and sexual assault can be very serious for everyone involved.

Legal consequences can include a prison sentence or criminal record, and being put on the sex offender register.

Being pressured to give consent

Physical and emotional consequences can last a lifetime.

Breaking the law

Consent is defined in law as "an agreement made by someone with the freedom and ability to decide something". Under the law, it is the person seeking consent who is responsible for ensuring that these conditions are met.

Sex without consent is rape or sexual abuse. Also, if you are a man forcing someone to perform oral sex on you, this is still rape. What's more, forcing someone into anal sex when they don't want to, even if that person has consented to vaginal sex, is still rape.

In the UK, people must be over 16 to legally consent to sex and they must be able to make informed decisions for themselves.

Advice on consent

How do I make sure I've got consent? How do I know if someone isn't giving consent?

Someone may confidently tell you upfront, or they may only show subtle body language that they're uncomfortable with the situation. Make sure you talk to your partner and that you're aware of the signs to spot around consent.

What can I do if my boyfriend or girlfriend wants me to do things that I'm not comfortable with?

If you don't want to do something sexual or have sex, it's absolutely OK to say or show that you don't want to, and the other person should stop.

Talk to your friends or someone you trust if you feel you are being forced to take part in sexual activity you don't want to.

What should you do if you're worried about a friend?

Sometimes your friends might not really understand consent or feel confident to seek it. If you hear them say things like "I didn't really want to, but…" it may mean they are being pressured by someone. It might help to ask if they want to talk about it.

The above information is reprinted with kind permission from DISRESPECT NOBODY.
© 2020 Crown copyright

www.disrespectnobody.co.uk

Online dating and staying safe

Seven million of us in the UK are registered with an online dating service, right now.

Healthy lives for young people

And it's not hard to understand why – it's an instantaneous, low-effort way to flirt and meet new people and we probably all know someone who met a partner online. In fact – it's how a quarter of us will meet our other half.

The vast majority of people using dating services are there with good, honest intentions. But what about the people that aren't?

At the risk of sounding like a killjoy, it's important to stop for a minute and make sure you're aware of the pitfalls and risks.

Here is our advice for using dating services safely:

Making contact

Watch what you share

One of the golden rules of online dating is don't exchange personal information. This starts with the username you pick; avoid something that might give something away about you, such as your surname, age or year of birth. Second, until you've met and feel you can trust the person you've met online, don't share your address, where you work or study, your phone number or email address.

Stay in the app

It's safer to keep using the messaging function within the dating app or site until you feel you have met and can trust them. If they ask for your number, or ask you to email them or switch to WhatsApp (a common trick among scammers is to say their subscription is running out), just politely decline and say it's nothing personal, it's just your policy not to.

Get to know them first. It can be a good idea to message and get to know a bit about each other before meeting up. It can help to give you a sense of who they are – and whether you have things in common. Just think about the details you're sharing about you and your life. Avoid saying exactly where you live and work for example, until you've got to know each other a bit better and feel you can trust them.

"My advice would be to not accept a date with someone straight after making contact"

"My advice would be to not accept a date with someone straight after making contact. I remember meeting someone on a dating site who asked me on a date straight after we matched. At the time I thought 'why not, what's the point in chatting for hours or even days, why waste time?'. But when we met, there was something about him that made me feel slightly uneasy. With hindsight, I'd say – try to have a conversation, get a feel for who they are, what their interests are, what they do for a living." – Anna

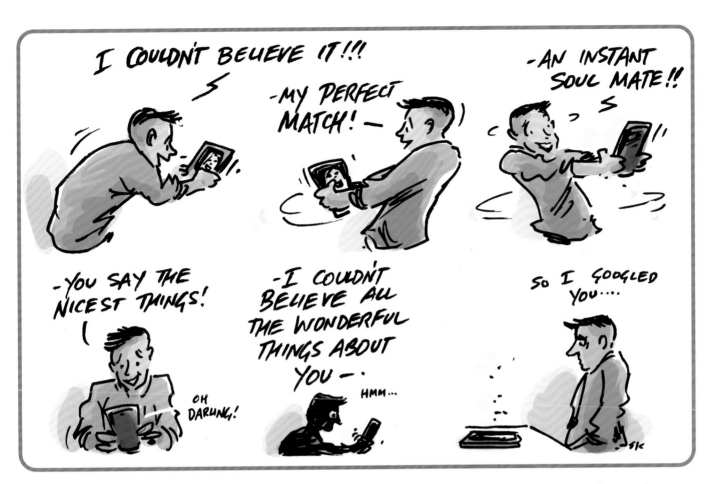

Apply a filter

Would you say the same things with someone face-to-face? If not, it's best not to online either.

Picture sharing

Whether it's your profile pictures or those sent to individuals you're chatting to, think before you share. Sharing naked or provocative images can attract attention that you may not be looking for and could lead to risky situations that are beyond your control.

"For some reason which escapes me now I put up relatively revealing pictures and an online handle ('Clare wants to play' – CRINGE!!) on one profile that weren't exactly designed to elicit a particularly mature response. Consequently I got lots of messages from people who I had no interest in, and looking back it was a risky thing to do because I invited unwanted attention." Clare

Google them

Try Googling what you know about them and do a Google image search to see where else their photo has appeared. Also, see if you have shared friends on Facebook or look them up on LinkedIn. That can be a great way to suss them out in advance. And trust us, this is not weird, stalk-y behavior. It's totally sensible and they're probably doing the same to you.

Trust your gut

Just like when you meet someone face-to-face, your instincts will tell you if something's not quite right. Maybe they won't tell you much about themselves but ask you a ton of questions, or perhaps they've declared their undying love you before you've even met. If it feels weird, chances are something's not what it seems. Trust your instincts and

be cautious until you've had long enough to really get to know someone. And if you're really not sure, run it by a friend that you trust to get some advice.

Consider the risks

Bear in mind that there's a limit to an online dating service's ability to do background checks or verify someone's identity. They can't, for instance, do criminal records checks on every user. Do as much research as you can, trust your judgement and make an informed decision before meeting up with someone.

Meeting up

Keep it casual

A good tip is to keep it super-casual. If you go for a coffee or a drink, it is much easier to end the date than if you've committed to a sit down meal. But by the same token, if it goes well, you can easily carry on and let it turn into lunch or dinner.

"One date was a disaster. I had no interest in the guy whatsoever, and the mature response would have been to have dinner (as planned), split the bill and go home. Instead I dealt with it by getting drunk and kissing him at a club. I vaguely remember he paid for everything. Thank god I didn't go home with him, but unsurprisingly he thought I liked him. When I got home and sobered up I felt pretty rubbish and wanted to put an end to the whole thing immediately, so I sent him a message thanking him for a lovely evening but that I didn't want to go on a second date. He did not take it. I got a very angry accusatory email accusing me of leading him on and the fact he'd paid all night definitely got mentioned. I then started to feel quite worried as we'd met not far from my work and I might have mentioned that I worked in the area… Luckily after a few bad emails I never heard from him again." Carrie

Go public

Another golden rule of dating is: always meet in a public place. Never meet at their house or invite them to yours and make sure it's a place where there are lots of people around and ideally – where you have phone signal. It is also a good idea to meet somewhere that you know well and are familiar with so you know how to get home.

"Make sure you meet in a busy place, a bar or pub. And try to arrange to meet somewhere in the middle that's easy for you to get home from." Anna

Tell a friend

Make sure that someone knows you're on a date and where you are. Also, try to text that friend if there's a change to the plan – or just to keep them updated about how it's going. You should also let them know when the date is over.

"I would text my friend regularly while I was on a date with someone I met online. You should make sure those close to you know where you are and what you're doing, at the very least." Clare

Stay charged

Make sure your phone is charged and that you have enough credit to call or text someone – you don't want to get caught short. And it's a good idea to keep your phone with you at all times.

Arrange your own transport

Letting your date collect you from or drop you off (especially at home) might not be a good idea. Think through your travel plans in advance and if they offer, you can thank them and say you'll make your own way. Also, try to meet somewhere that you can get back from easily.

Long distance dates

If you live some distance from one another, you need to take extra care if you travel to meet them. Stay in a hotel or B&B and keep the location private. If they want to pick you up or walk you back to where you're staying, you could also say you're staying somewhere else. And if you can't afford to stay in a hotel, you shouldn't go. You might feel like you really know them and have built a bond but agreeing to stay with them is not wise either.

Watch your stuff

Most of us will rely on a bit of Dutch courage to get through a date but keep it to a level that you're under control and don't leave your drink unattended. Also, don't leave your phone, wallet or bags unattended. Keep them with you at all times.

Feeling uncomfortable?

Leave at any time if you feel uncomfortable, your safety is the most important thing. If you feel embarrassed or guilty about leaving, tell them you feel unwell and make your excuses. Or text a friend and get them to ring you and pretend they need you.

"My advice would be – never feel like you have to stay out with someone if you're not interested in them."

"I realised pretty quickly after meeting him that there was no connection. Out of all the dates I'd been on there was something about this man that made me feel slightly uneasy. But I was polite so stayed out for a couple of hours and then went home. The next day I told him (in the nicest way) that I was not interested. His initial response was polite and accepting but about an hour later I received quite an angry message from him that left me with an uncomfortable feeling, I'd never experienced that sort of response from other men I'd met online. I didn't respond and I deleted him straight away. My advice would be – never feel like you have to stay out with someone if you're not interested in them – just to be polite. There's nothing wrong with ending a date early and going home." Hannah

Things you should report

Requests for money

Dating services work hard to stamp this sort of thing out but be mindful of the fact that if someone asks you for money, they're almost certainly a scammer. They might tell you they need to buy a plane or train ticket, that they're widowed, that their relative is sick or that they will give you something in return. Whatever the story, never ever give out your bank details or give someone money and if they ask, stop replying and report them immediately to protect both you and others from being scammed. If you've already done this, report it immediately through Action Fraud.

Offensive, insulting or threatening messages

If you feel sure you're talking to someone who isn't who they say they are, or if they're threatening, offensive or insulting, report it to the dating site or app you're using. Don't feel embarrassed or like you're wasting their time. You're helping them keep their site safe and before you brush it off as being a bad experience, just think about the next person they get chatting to. Dating sites and apps usually take their members' safety seriously and will have in-built features to block or report.

Obscene images

If you receive obscene, pornographic, violent or abusive images via a dating service, report it to the dating site and the police immediately. Depending on the content, this is likely to be illegal.

The above information is reprinted with kind permission from Brook.
©2020 Brook Young People

www.brook.org.uk

What is sexting?

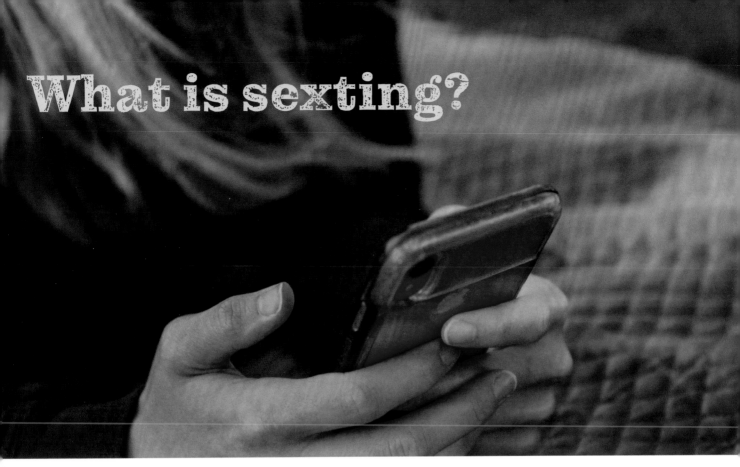

Sexting is when someone sends or receives a sexually explicit text, image or video. This includes sending 'nude pics', 'rude pics' or 'nude selfies'. Pressuring someone into sending a nude pic can happen in any relationship and to anyone, whatever their age, gender or sexual preference.

It's easy to think that everybody is sending these nude selfies – they're not! Putting pressure on someone to send a nude pic, or sharing someone's picture without their permission, even if it's a friend and they say it's just banter, is wrong and even illegal.

Signs you're being pressured to sext

How are people pressured into sending pics?

♦ Made to feel like everyone is doing it

♦ Called names like 'frigid' to bully them into sending one

♦ Emotional pressure so they feel guilty if they don't want to. This can include being told things like 'if you loved me you would' or 'I sent you one so you owe me'

♦ Threatened with consequences if they don't. For example, threatening to 'out' someone as gay or bi-sexual if they don't send a pic, or threatening to spread rumours about someone.

It's never OK to pressure someone into sexting and you always have the right to say no. Even if it's with someone you're in a relationship with (sexual or not) and even if you have done it before.

Potential consequences of sexting

What does the law say?

Taking, possessing or sharing a sexually explicit picture or video of someone under 18 is against the law. It doesn't matter if they gave you permission, someone else sent it to you, you've never met them before, you are under 18 too or it's a selfie. You and anyone else involved could be investigated by the police, and this could even affect your future education and employment.

If you are over 18 and you send an image of yourself to someone who is also over 18, this is not a crime. However, you should consider the other consequences of sending and sharing images.

'Once it's gone, it's gone'

When you share a picture or video online or on your phone, you lose control of it. Pictures can be quickly shared over the internet. Once somebody else has it they can send it to anyone. Think how you'd feel if your nude selfie was sent to your friends, family or teachers, or if you were involved in forwarding a 'sext' of someone under 18 that results in a police investigation.

Feeling pressured to send pics can affect your confidence

If someone is pressuring you to send a nude pic this is wrong. It's a form of abuse and can damage your confidence and self-worth.

You could be blackmailed

If you send a picture you wouldn't want other people to see, then you could be in danger of being blackmailed. The person who received it might threaten to share the photo unless you send them more. If you are gay or bi-sexual, this could include threatening to 'out' you, or you could experience homophobic or bi-phobic bullying, along with the humiliation of the image being shared. If you're exploring your sexuality or gender, you can get advice from a trusted organisation like Stonewall.

Pressuring someone to send an image

If you're pressuring someone to send you sexually explicit or nude pictures, this is abusive and not normal or acceptable. If they are under 18 it's illegal to take, possess or share an indecent image.

What about forwarding on a pic someone has sent you?

Don't share anyone else's nude pictures. If you forward a nude or sexually explicit picture or video of someone without their consent, you're breaking the law and taking part in abuse that could cause them serious distress.

Frequently asked questions about sexting

I've been asked to send a nude pic – what should I do?

It can be really stressful when you don't want to send a nude pic but you don't want to be bullied for not sending one either. It's important to know that lots of people have been in this situation before and help and support is available. Childline offers some great tips, like giving you killer comebacks using its ZIPIT app when someone is pressuring you for a pic.

What can I do if someone is threatening to share photos of me?

If someone is threatening to send your nude picture to others then they are committing a serious crime and the best thing to do is get help.

Don't give in to threats. Walk away and tell an adult you trust. If you think you are in immediate danger call 999. If your pictures are being used against you then you can report it to CEOP (Child Exploitation and Online Protection Centre). They help young people who are being targeted online or suffering sexual abuse.

What can I do if someone shares a pic I sent them?

It can be upsetting to find out someone has done this but there are things you can do. Tell someone you trust as soon as possible, such as a parent, guardian or teacher, so they can take action and try to stop the image being shared further. It may be embarrassing but remember you are not the first person this has happened to and your school will have ways of dealing with this.

Childline and Thinkuknow offer lots of practical advice and support, such as how to request for images to be removed from some sites.

Should you send pictures to someone you've only met online?

Remember that people you are in contact with online may not be who they say they are or even be the same age as you. If someone you've met online is putting pressure on you to send sexual images of yourself or do sexual things on webcam, you can report it to CEOP who can help stop this. Visit Childline and CEOP for more advice about sexting and online safety and if you are immediate danger, call 999.

If you're lesbian, gay, bisexual or transgender sometimes it might seem easier to meet other LGB&T people online, especially if you're not out, and it can be hard when other people you know are starting relationships but you haven't. But sending nude pics to somebody you don't know can be dangerous. There might be an LGB&T group in your local area where you could meet other young LGB&T people in confidence, supported by a professional adult.

What should you do if you're worried about a friend?

If your friend is worried about sexting and saying things to you like 'I didn't really want to send it but…', they might need help.

Talk to them and let them know where they can get help.

Is it OK to ask someone for a nude pic if you're going out with them?

If somebody doesn't want to send a nude pic, it's really important that you accept that and don't try to change their mind. Pressuring somebody into sending a nude pic is wrong and there can be serious consequences.

And don't forget that if someone is under 18 it's illegal for them to send pics of themselves and for you to possess them.

My mates keep pressuring me to get a nude pic of someone but I don't want to, what can I do?

It's wrong to pressure anyone to do something they don't want to do. Some people see having nude pics on their phone as a status symbol, but they may have pressured others to send them the photos. If your mates are pressuring you to do this it is wrong and it is abusive behaviour. Also, if someone is under 18 it's illegal for them to send nude or sexually explicit pics of themselves and for you to possess or share them.

The above information is reprinted with kind permission from DISRESPECT NOBODY.
© 2020 Crown copyright

www.disrespectnobody.co.uk

All St Andrews University students to have 'sexual consent lessons' after claims of rape and sex assault

All St Andrews students are to be given compulsory lessons on sexual consent after the Fife university was rocked by allegations of rape and sexual assault.

According to the Daily Telegraph, at least nine rape claims were made against students in Alpha Epsilon Pi, a global fraternity with 'chapters' across the globe. The St Andrews chapter consists of about 50 men.

Allegations were also made on Instagram account St Andrews Survivors, which last week began sharing anonymous accounts of sexual misconduct at the university.

Not all claims shared by the page relate to incidents at the university, with some predating students' time at St Andrews.

Alpha Epsilon Pi (AEPi) has vowed to suspend the members accused and include "mandatory consent education and anti-rape culture education" in new member and chapter programmes.

"We find the content of these allegations abhorrent and we take them extremely seriously," the fraternity said in a statement.

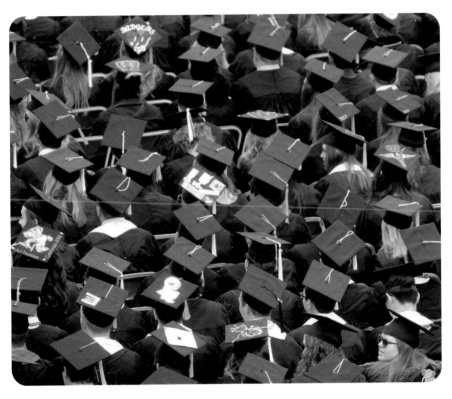

"The fraternity unconditionally opposes, and its conditions of membership absolutely prohibit, any conduct considered sexual harassment or sexual assault."

The university is to introduce a "compulsory orientation module" for the upcoming academic year which will require students to learn more about consent and sexual assault before arriving. All students will be required to complete the course online.

A spokeswoman for the university said: "We welcome the 'St Andrews Survivors' account's efforts to provide people of all genders a space to voice their experiences of sexual misconduct.

"The Proctor met with the account creator this week to establish how we can work together to signpost support and reporting mechanisms to students who require them.

"It is categorically untrue to suggest the university tried to suppress survivor testimonies, as the account creator has made clear.

"The university's primary concern is to ensure survivors know that we are ready and willing to support their decisions and take action, facilitate police reporting, and provide ongoing support accordingly.

"We appreciate these are difficult issues to speak about, but our student services team has a 90% satisfaction rating amongst students, and survivors who wish to see perpetrators investigated must be willing to make reports through the appropriate channels.

"We have clear and established procedures for investigating allegations of this nature.

"However, the details of any investigations must remain confidential to offer appropriate support and fair outcomes to all concerned. It would not be appropriate for us to comment on whether any specific individual or group is under investigation.

"The university will always act when incidents are formally reported, and is committed to working collaboratively with students to promote a culture of responsibility and respect, in which everyone can trust in our procedures and that our community is intolerant of all forms of sexual misconduct."

Yvonne Stenhouse, Police Scotland's community inspector for North East Fife, said:

"We are aware of these online reports and are working with the university."

11 July 2020

The above information is reprinted with kind permission from DC THOMSON MEDIA.
© DC Thomson Co Ltd 2020.

www.thecourier.co.uk

Why we need to talk to young people about pornography

It's no surprise that developments in technology have revolutionised the way we carry out almost every aspect of our daily lives. From the first email being sent in the 1970s, the introduction of the World Wide Web in 1991, and the first ever mobile phone with internet connectivity launching in 1996, we've come a long way. Hello, Google!

Much of the way we use technology is of course amazing and has enriched our lives for the better. We can stay connected, have access to a world of knowledge, and create totally new ways of doing things. However, the development of technology has also impacted upon our young people in one aspect more negatively than any other – the introduction of free, easily accessible online pornography.

A digital society

The majority of teens and 'tweens' (those aged 9-12) own a smartphone and are using social media platforms such as Instagram and Snapchat on a daily basis. Especially if you are a parent, you'll know this means your children ultimately have 24/7 access to billions of websites and social media accounts in the palm of their hands — including pornography.

In culture where smartphones keep this abundance of content constantly available to young people, and where social media has become intrinsic to many of their lives, young people are growing up in a world inundated by selfies, where they feel a pressure to constantly share 'life updates' and images of themselves, and hence compare themselves to others.

Research by Hugues and Rosamund in 2015 suggests that young people who are heavy users of social media – spending more than two hours per day on social networking sites such as Facebook, Twitter or Instagram – are more likely to report poor mental health, including psychological distress (symptoms of anxiety and depression).

Free, online streaming of pornography is currently not regulated in the UK – meaning anyone can access one of the thousands of sites on the web – and with the development of smartphones, young people are seeing pornographic and sexually explicit content on their social media accounts.

The NSPCC found that children are as likely to stumble across pornography accidentally as they are to search for it or be shown it by someone else, while GirlGuiding found that 60% of girls aged 11-21 say that they see boys their age viewing pornography on mobile devices such as phones or tablets, often while at school.

60% of girls aged 11-21 say they see boys their age viewing pornography on mobile devices

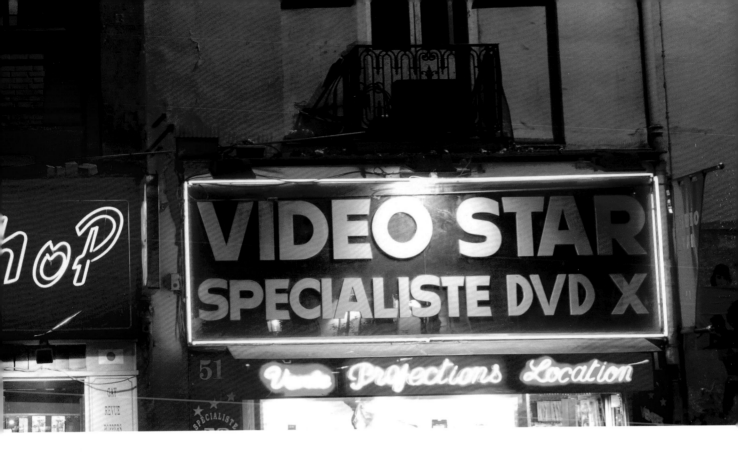

Where are children learning about sex?

Without effective education on pornography, sexual consent and healthy relationships, many young people are left to seek out education on sex from pornography.

What this means is that their developing brains, particularly young boys who are the main viewers of pornography, are exposed to a plethora of unrealistic and in many cases increasingly violent content. In an analysis of over 300 scenes of pornography, one study found that almost 90% contained some form of physical aggression, predominantly by a man against a woman. Targets of this aggression showed pleasure or responded neutrally.

A report published by the National Union of Students (NUS) found that 60% of students surveyed use pornography to find out more about sex, with three quarters agreeing it provided unrealistic expectations. Young people, without formal education, are not able to understand the complexity of the pornography industry, and that the content they are seeing is not real, nor is it a lesson on what sex should look like.

GirlGuiding's study found that 71% of girls aged 17-21 think that pornography gives out confusing messages about sexual consent, and the same amount think it makes aggressive behaviour towards women seem normal. This is extremely worrying, as it means many young women and men are growing up with a distorted idea about what they can expect when it comes to sex and intimacy.

What needs to change?

We must call on the government to ensure that all children and young people receive a rounded, informative and empowering age-appropriate sex and relationship education (SRE) throughout their time at school and college. Currently, only pupils attending local-authority run secondary schools, which represent around a third of secondary schools, are offered sex and relationships education.

A revised SRE curriculum is not set to be introduced in schools now until September 2020, and parents are only obligated for their children to attend a limited part of the education; all other parts they can withdraw their children from.

We strongly believe that children and young people deserve, and require, a holistic education on issues around sexual consent, pornography, online safety, healthy relationships and domestic abuse; an education which does not only exist in schools, but in their families, communities, college, universities and beyond.

Parents are pivotal in this education, as they can give their children the information they need to understand the potentially harmful effects of pornography, social media and the internet.

By speaking openly with young people about the issues they may very well face, we can better support them to make educated, healthy decisions about their own lives and to take care of those around them – skills which will stay with them throughout their entire adult lives.

20 July 2018

The above information is reprinted with kind permission from UK SAYS NO MORE.
©2020 UK SAYS NO MORE

www.uksaysnomore.org

Key Facts

- Being sexually healthy is about having safe and respectful relationships, and not having to do anything sexually that you don't want to. Being emotionally OK is a really important part of sexual health too. This means feeling good about your sexual experiences, and not regretting anything that's happened. (page 1)

- Apart from abstaining from sex, condoms are the most effective method to prevent STIs. However, they are not 100% effective and do not cover the whole genital area. It is possible to catch some infections including Herpes and Syphilis through skin-on-skin contact alone. (page 3)

- There are 2 human papillomavirus (HPV) vaccination programmes in the UK. One is for children who are 12 to 13 years of age, and one is for men who have sex with men (MSM) up to 45 years of age. (page 5)

- In the 1960s, only 1% of girls would enter puberty before their ninth birthday. Today, up to 40% of some populations in both rich and poor countries are doing so. (page 6)

- Periods are still treated as a taboo subject in many parts of the world. Despite being a completely normal biological function, they are often seen as shameful, embarrassing and impure. (page 10)

- "Chhaupadi" is a practice common in Nepal where during menstruation, women and girls must must sleep outside the family home, traditionally in a purpose built menstrual hut, known as a "chhau goth". This practice was officially criminalised in August 2018. (page 10)

- Of the 1.9 billion women of reproductive age (15-49 years) worldwide in 2019, 1.1 billion had a need for family planning; of these, 842 million used contraceptive methods, and 270 million had an unmet need for contraception. (page 11)

- Sexual health budgets of local councils have been slashed by £55.7m since 2013/14. (page14)

- According to Public Health England figures published in 2018, 447,694 sexually transmitted infections (STIs) were reported in England. (page 15)]

- Globally, more than 30% of all new HIV infections occur in young people aged 15 to 25, according to the World Health Organization (WHO). (page 16)

- Today, more than five million young people live with HIV, according to the WHO. (page 16)

- The number of new HIV diagnoses in the UK has fallen by almost a third since 2015 and is at its lowest level since 2000, figures by Public Health England have revealed. (page 18)

- Data has shown there were 4,484 new diagnoses of HIV in 2018 compared to 6,271 in 2015 – a decline of 28%. (page 18)

- Between 2014 and 2018 there was a 13.9% increase in new STI diagnoses in men aged 45-64. There was also a 23% increase in diagnoses amongst both men and women aged 65+. (page 19)

- The most commoinly diagnosed STIs on 2018 were:
  - chlamydia (49% of all new diagnoses)
  - first episode genital warts (13%)
  - gonorrhoea (13%)
  - first episode genital herpes (8%). (page 20)

- By 2058, the National HPV Immunisation programme could prevent up to 64,138 HPV-related cervical cancers and almost 50,000 other HPV-related cancers. (page 20)

- Sexually transmitted infections (STIs) are any kind of bacterial or viral infection that can be passed on through unprotected sexual contact. They can have a number of signs and symptoms; however, some STIs have no symptoms, and if left untreated can lead to infertility. (page 23)

- Contraception and sexual health services such as Brook are free and confidential, including for people under the age of 16. (page 23)

- Most STIs can be easily treated with antibiotics. (page 25)

- Consent has to be given freely and no one can be made to consent to something. It's not consent if someone does something because they feel like they have to. You can also never assume that someone is giving consent – you have to be sure. (page 31)

- Taking, possessing or sharing a sexually explicit picture or video of someone under 18 is against the law. It doesn't matter if they gave you permission, someone else sent it to you, you've never met them before, you are under 18 too or it's a selfie. You and anyone else involved could be investigated by the police, and this could even affect your future education and employment. (page 35)

- GirlGuiding found that 60% of girls aged 11-21 say that they see boys their age viewing pornography on mobile devices such as phones or tablets, often while at school. (page 38)

- A report published by the National Union of Students (NUS) found that 60% of students surveyed use pornography to find out more about sex, with three quarters agreeing it provided unrealistic expectations. (page 39)

Cervical cancer

Cancer that develops in a woman's cervix (the entrance to the womb from the vagina). In its early stages it often has no symptoms. Symptoms can include unusual vaginal bleeding which can occur after sex, in between periods or after menopause. The NHS offers a national screening programmw, a 'smear test' for all women between the ages of 25 and 64 years old.

Condoms

A thin rubber (latex) sleeve worn on the penis. When used correctly, condoms are the only form of contraception that protect against pregnancy and STIs. They are 98% effective – this means that two out of 100 women using male condoms as contraception will become pregnant in one year. You can get free condoms from sexual health clinics and some GP surgeries.

Contraception

Anything which prevents conception, or pregnancy, from taking place. 'Barrier methods', such as condoms, work by stopping sperm from reaching an egg during intercourse and are also effective in preventing STIs. Hormonal methods such as the contraceptive pill change the way a woman's body works to prevent an egg from being fertilised.

Contraceptive implant

A small flexible tube about the size of a matchstick inserted by a doctor under the skin of the female's upper arm. The device releases hormones to prevent the ovaries from releasing eggs. Lasts for three years, but can be removed before then if the woman decide she wants to get pregnant.

Contraceptive injections

An injection offers eight to 12 weeks protection against pregnancy, but not from sexually transmitted diseases (approx 99% effective). It works by thickening the mucus in the cervix, which stops sperm reaching the egg, and it also thins the lining of the womb so that an egg can't implant itself there.

Diaphragms

A rubber dome-shaped device worn inside the vagina which creates a seal against the walls of the vagina, It must be inserted before sexual intercourse and must remain in place for up to six to eight hours afterwards. The diaphragnm does not provide protection from STIs.

Emergency contraception

Emergency contraception, commonly known as the 'morning after pill', is used after unprotected sex to prevent a fertilised egg from becoming implanted in the womb. It can be taken by females within 72 hrs after unprotected sex (although preferably within the first 24 hours). It should not be used as a regular method of contraception. It is available across the counter at chemists or from your local GP or sexual health clinic.

Female condom

Sometimes known as a femidom, a female condom is worn inside the vagina during sex to prevent pregnancy. They're a barrier method of contraception, protecting against pregnancy as well as STIs. If used correctly they are 95% effective.

HPV vaccination

The vaccine is effective at stopping people getting the high-risk types of HPV that cause cancer, including most cervical cancers and some anal, genital, mouth and throat (head and neck) cancers. In England, all boys and girls aged 12 to 13 years are routinely offered the 1st HPV vaccination when they're in Year 8 at school. The 2nd dose is offered 6 to 24 months after the 1st dose.

Safe sex

Being safe with sex means caring for your own health and the health of your partner. Being safe protects you from getting or passing on STIs and from unplanned pregnancy.

Sexual health

Taking care of your sexual health means more than being free from STIs or not having to face an unplanned pregnancy. It also means taking responsibility for your body, your health, your partner's health and your decisions about sex.

Sexually transmitted infections

An infection that is transmitted through sexual contact and the exchange of bodily fluids such as semen.

The pill

A tablet taken each day, at the same time, by girls to prevent pregnancy. The pill contains hormones that prevent ovaries from releasing an egg. It only protects against pregnancy and not STIs.

Activities

Brainstorming

- What is included in the term 'sexual health'?

- In pairs, list as many myths about sexual health as you can think of.

- What kind of sexual health services are available in your local area?

- In small groups, create a mind-map of all the things that you can do take care of yourself and your sexual health.

Research

- Do some online research and share your findings on two of the following methods of contraception:
  - Male condom
  - The pill
  - IUD
  - WIthdrawal

- Conduct an anonymous questionnaire to find out what your peers think about sex education in your school. You should aim to find out whether they think it is useful, up-to-date and appropriate. You should also aim to find out whether there is anything your peers think should be covered at school that, currently, is not. When you have gathered your results, write a report that summarises your findings. Include graphs and tables.

- Choose a country in Europe (apart from the UK) and research its laws and policies regarding sexual health and sex education. How do they compare to this country? Write a short paragraph explaining what you've found.

- Using the internet, look at UK news stories from the last year where there have been court hearings about the issue of consent in rape cases. How many can you find, what were the outcomes and what are the main similarities between the cases?

Design

- Choose one of the articles from this book and create an illustration that highlights the key themes of the piece.

- Design a poster that could be displayed in a local GP's office explaining the risks of STIs and how to prevent them.

- Create an informative leaflet about the different kinds of sexually transmitted infections, how they are transmitted and the treatment options available for each.

- In small groups, design a storyboard for a series of YouTube videos that will promote the use of contraception among young people.

- Draw a cartoon strip about how to use a condom correctly that would be suitable to be used in an RSE lesson for your age group.

Oral

- In pairs, discuss the definitions of :
  - consent
  - sexting

- Chlamydia is the most common sexually transmitted infection among young people. Create an informative presentation on the signs and symptoms of chlamydia, the risks associated with it and how it can be treated.

- As a class, discuss whether you think pornography should be shown as part of sex education lessons.

- At what age should sex education be taught? How young is too young? Debate this as a group.

- In small groups, explore the qualities of good and bad relationships. After discussion, make a list of the best qualities and a list of the worst qualities.

Reading/writing

- Write a one-paragraph definition of the term 'sexual health' and compare with a classmate's.

- Imagine that you represent a UK charity that offers advice and support on all matters of sexual wellbeing. Compose a selection of social media posts for Twitter, Facebook and Instagram aimed at making young people aware of the importance of sexual health and practising safe sex. You may also post links to external websites, videos and photos which provide further information if you think this is helpful.

- What is the definition of rape? Look at sex and the law in the UK. What are the possible consequences of sex or physical closeness without consent? Consider not just the legal impact, the health and emotional effects, too. Write a summary of your findings.

- Sexual health is not just all about STIs, it is also about a respectful understanding of sex, relationships and the mental and emotional aspects involved. Make a list of all the things a person should consider before having sexual intercourse.

Acknowledgements

The publisher is grateful for permission to reproduce the material in this book. While every care has been taken to trace and acknowledge copyright, the publisher tenders its apology for any accidental infringement or where copyright has proved untraceable. The publisher would be pleased to come to a suitable arrangement in any such case with the rightful owner.

The material reproduced in *ISSUES* books is provided as an educational resource only. The views, opinions and information contained within reprinted material in *ISSUES* books do not necessarily represent those of Independence Educational Publishers and its employees.

Images

Cover image courtesy of iStock. All other images courtesy of Pixabay and Unsplash, except pages 38-39: iStock.

Illustrations

Simon Kneebone: pages 3, 24 & 33. Angelo Madrid: page 20 & 30.

Additional acknowledgements

With thanks to the Independence team: Shelley Baldry, Danielle Lobban, Jackie Staines and Jan Sunderland.

Tracy Biram

Cambridge, September 2020